Be Healthier

Be Healthier

Start Your Own Journey Today

Mohd Ilhan Abdullah

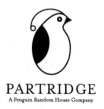

PARTRIDGE
A Penguin Random House Company

To order additional copies of this book, contact
Toll Free 800 101 2657 (Singapore)
Toll Free 1 800 81 7340 (Malaysia)
orders.singapore@partridgepublishing.com

www.partridgepublishing.com/singapore

Acknowledgements

I wish to express my gratitude to all the gracious and wonderful people who have

- written books,
- contributed articles,
- created websites and blogs, and
- posted videos

in the fields of

- human physiology,
- health and wellness,
- food and nutrition,
- exercise, and
- rest and recreation.

Their willingness to share their information, knowledge, expertise and experience is truly magnanimous and deeply appreciated by all those seeking to be healthier.

May all their good work continue and may they find all that they seek.

Contents

Appendices

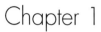

Chapter 1

Change Begins With Me

Introduction

In the 21st Century, there has been a big jump in the number of people suffering from diseases like obesity, diabetes, high blood pressure, acid reflux. The incidences of stroke and heart attack have also gone up accordingly.

Previously, people thought that these non-communicable diseases were "rich men's diseases"; the poor rarely suffered from such. But this is no more the case; rich and poor, young and old are equally afflicted today.

For these people with any one of the afflictions, quality of life has taken a knock as dependence on medicine to get through the day has gone way, way up.

If you are amongst them, why are you not doing something about it? Is it because of one of the following reasons?

1. I have no time.
2. I do not know how.
3. I have tried before and failed.
4. Getting healthy is expensive.
5. It is too difficult.

My objectives in putting my thoughts on paper are to:

- share with you the information that I have;
- give you enough *basic* information and examples for you to understand what goes on inside your body;
- show you the food options that are available to you;

- motivate you to do the simple things to get healthier;
- help you to pluck the low-lying fruits straight away - simply, easily, economically.

This book is meant for beginners, those who are not feeling healthy and who want to take the first baby steps to better health. It is also for those who are rushed for time every day and desire to do something to help themselves within the time constraints that govern their lives.

This book is **NOT** meant for those who are already healthy and fit but who would like to be healthier and fitter than the normal person next door. There are many other good guides available for these fitness buffs.

You may well ask "what is required"? The time that is asked is minimal; the methods proposed are simple, easy and economical. You can be healthier in relatively quick time and at a very affordable cost.

The main requirement is to have faith in yourself and to make the commitment to yourself.

Faith + Commitment = Effort

"For things to change, I must change.
For things to get better, I must get better".
- Jim Rohn

Chapter 2

The More Things Change, The More They Stay The Same

Introduction

When I was in school (from the early 1950's through to 1965), I studied World History in the 1960's. I learnt that we once lived in caves; we hunted and foraged for food. We learnt how to use tools to hunt and gather. To survive, we depended on our physical prowess. In other words, the human body was, and still is, made for movement and activity.

Then came the Agricultural Revolution. Humans learnt to make use of the land to grow crops for food. They tilled the land, planted crops and harvested the fruits of their labour.

They also domesticated animals to give food. Hunting and foraging became less and less important. But there was still this reliance on physical capabilities.

During the Industrial Revolution that followed, humans moved away from the land into the cities to work in factories. In the era of mass production in factories, they used their labour to earn their upkeep. They began to rely less on the land for their livelihood. Dependence on physical labour grew less.

We are now in the Information Age where knowledge is key. Robotics. Process automation. Smart tools and gadgets. We have moved further away from labour and land to machines and now to use of the brain.

In terms of pleasurable pursuits, this trend has also been the same – less physical, more cerebral. Lifestyles have changed from much robust physical activity to one of sedentary pursuits.

The result - the human body, made for movement and physical activity - has fallen into greater disuse with the passage of time.

It took the Western world hundreds of years to shift from the age of hunting to the Agricultural Revolution. Then came another longish period to the Industrial Revolution. Now we are in the Information Age.

I have seen this evolution in the last 60 years in my own country, beginning in the 1950's. In the 1950's, my country was an agricultural economy. But in the space of about 60 years (1950's to 2010's) we have marched from agriculture to industrial to a service economy. Along the way, so many things have changed.

Conditions 60 Years Ago

Back in the 1950's and 1960's when I was growing up, the living conditions in Malaysia where I live were different. This was the era of the night soil carriers or the "bucket brigade". Sanitary conditions were not that modern then. Yet I dare say that the living conditions then made it easier to be healthy.

For starters, most things that needed to be done – housework, washing clothes, preparing food for the table, etc. – needed "elbow grease". In simple terms, it needed manual labour. There were no washing machines, no dish dryers, no food processors.

We washed clothes by hand, then hung them out to dry on bamboo poles in the open. We sliced and diced the food by hand before cooking. Cooking utensils, crockery and cutlery were all washed by hand and dried by hand. If anything needed to be pounded, there was the faithful pestle and mortar – made out of granite too! If any spices needed to be ground into paste, there was the grind stone – a flat granite slab and its granite rolling pin. Believe me when I say that granite rolling pins are heavy. See what I mean by "elbow grease"?

Back then, to go somewhere, there was the trustworthy Shank's Pony i.e. you walked. If you could afford it, you rode a bicycle. Or else took a bus. The wealthier folks had their little 50 cc motor bikes (Honda Cubs, no less); the even wealthier folks drove their cars (black Morris Minors, no less). But by and large it was Shank's Pony or the bicycle.

A lot of time was spent outdoors, playing childhood games which required physical activity. Television (black and white) was a luxury – and transmission was only for a few hours each night. There were no electronic gadgets – no tablets (only medicinal types around then), no iPads (just blackboards and chalk), no mobile phones (just land lines).

What about food? It was home cooking most of the time. Eating out was a treat – or when the ladies of the house decided that they did not wish to cook for that day. There were no McDonald's, no Kentucky Fried Chicken, no pizza joints and no donuts. Eating out was just eating somebody else's cooking for a change.

Lifestyle Changes – Last 60 Years

Over the last 60 years, many countries have made economic progress. Many families have benefitted from the economic progress of their respective countries. With economic progress has come lifestyle changes. These changes have impacted our health in many ways and continue to do so.

Today, physical activity has declined to a great extent and many a meal is made up of fast food - McDonald's or KFC or pizzas. This change did not happen overnight; it has crept up on us slowly but surely.

Today, people are less inclined to physical activity. In my neighbourhood, I still walk to the shops to get what I want. Be there and back within 15 minutes by the famous Shank's Pony. Just a little sweat but definitely no stress. Yet I know of neighbours who take the car, drive round the block of shops a few times just to find a parking space, get the stuff that they came for and drive home. 30 minutes all told – no sweat but much stress from traffic and trying to find parking space. Sounds familiar?

Running late – for reasons beyond your control. No time to prepare food at home. Just pop into the nearest fast food place and buy some food. Alternatively, get home first and order some food for home delivery - Mac's or KFC or pizza. Add-on the soda, energy/sport drinks and dessert – rich and sweet. Good to eat, fills the stomach but not enough nutritional value.

Another phenomenon – in my own country no less – is the proliferation of 24-hour eateries. These have sprung up like mushrooms and they are constantly crowded too – any time of day and night. And we wonder why so many more people are overweight and not too healthy!

This combination of *reduced physical activity* and *changes in our dietary habits* has made more people unhealthy than ever before.

The Human Body

Over the centuries, no matter what has changed in the external environment, there has been one constant – the human body. Its make-up has remained the same; how it functions has not altered at all.

There is no doubt that in the coming years, more change in the external world will materialise. It does not matter where you live – China, or the Middle East, or Eastern Europe. Economic progress will impact your country. More countries will be on the same path, shifting from an agricultural economy to an industrial one and then on to a service and knowledge-based economy.

In the course of this economic transition, living standards are going to go up; living conditions are going to improve; lifestyle is going to change. More and more people will experience these changes, at a faster rate even.

So do be prepared to take advantage of economic advancement and prosperity coming your way. Just remember this –you must remain healthy to pursue your dreams and enjoy the benefits that follow.

My one wish for you – STAY HEALTHY.

To do so, it is important that you know more about the human body and how it functions.

Chapter 3

Cells and Cellular Nutrition

The Human Body

The human body is a living, breathing organism. The smallest unit of life that is in the human body is the *cell.*

A group of similar cells that perform a particular function makes up a type of *tissue.* For example, nervous tissue is made up of nerve cells. Other examples are the smooth muscle tissue and cardiac tissue.

Two or more types of tissue that work together to perform one or more body functions make up an *organ.* Examples of organs are the brain, the heart, the lungs, the liver, the kidneys, etc. I am sure that you can name many more.

Every organ is part of one or more of the body's total of 12 *specialised systems which make up the human body.* 11 of these systems help us to sustain life; 1 specialised system is for procreation.

As humans, we are all blessed with the same structure and systems.

The important principles to grasp here are: –

- *The human body is made up of cells; a cell is the fundamental building block of life.*
- *Cells multiply (divide themselves)*
- *As cells mature, they turn into specialised cells carrying out specialised functions.*

- *Cells make tissues, tissues make up organs, organs make up systems, and systems make up the human body.*

Cell Regeneration

Cells grow and divide; older cells die, leaving the younger cells to regenerate yet younger cells. And so the cycle of cell regeneration goes.

All cells do not divide and mature at the same rate. Some cells regenerate in days, some in months, yet others over years. For example, the cells lining our stomach regenerate over 5 days – they need to because of the acid that they are exposed to in the stomach. Skin cells regenerate in three months. Red blood cells live for 4 months; the cells of the liver live for 5 months. In terms of longevity, a bone takes about 10 years or so to completely replace itself. Cells in the intestines live for about 15 years. There are some really important cells in your body that do not regenerate or do so very slowly —those of your bones, your brain, and your heart.

What does this regeneration of cells mean? It means that at any one time, the organs in the body have a mix of young cells and older cells. The key issue here is – are the younger cells healthier than the older cells which they are replacing? If the answer is yes, then you will have a predominance of healthy, younger cells. What it means is that you can grow healthier over time.

If your younger cells are not as healthy as the older ones which are dying off, you will end up with a predominance of unhealthier younger cells which will divide into more of the same cells if you do not take action to be healthier. Over the course of time, your health will deteriorate.

In the context of health,

- *healthy cells regenerate healthy cells;*
- *healthy cells means healthy tissues, healthy tissues make up healthy organs, healthy organs make up healthy systems. Healthy systems make up a healthy body.*
- *In contrast, unhealthy cells reproduce unhealthy cells, leading to unhealthy tissues, organs and body systems.*

Cellular Nutrition

A living organism, whether it be plant, animal or human, needs nutrients for it to survive. The organism will survive if it gets these nutrients in the minimum quantity. Getting the optimum quantity will enable the organism to not only survive but thrive. What, then, are the essential needs of the human body?

Different body cells need different nutrients in differing quantity. Not only that, there are combinations of nutrients that make sure that an organ functions to the best of its ability. At its most fundamental, it means eating food that has the nutrition needed by the cells in the body.

In essence, the body needs an energy source (usually from the food group carbohydrates), 8 essential amino acids (proteins) for building muscles, 13 vitamins, 21 minerals and 2 essential fatty acids (EFA's). If you get sufficient quantities of these nutrients, the cells will get all the nutrients needed.

It is your responsibility to eat what your cells need, not what tastes good and fills you up only. If you eat all kinds of food devoid of the nutrients needed by your body, there will be consequences over the long term.

So what is the importance of eating right? Simply put, good food makes your immune system stronger; your energy levels are higher; you are fitter and more active. Maintaining a healthy weight is easier. Your skin complexion is better. You concentrate better; you do not get irritated as easily; your cells grow - and damaged cells regrow - healthily.

If you feed your cells what they need, you will be rewarded with better health over the long term.

"Understand that you have the ability to get healthy and stay healthy."

Dr. Christiane Northrup

Chapter 4

Body Systems

Systems of the Human Body

The Organ Systems

Your body is made up of 11 organ systems that help you to survive and 1 organ system that helps you to preserve the human race.

Within each organ system (or community),

- there are individual organs that perform specific tasks;
- the individual organs work with other organs within the specific system;
- each system also works with other systems to help you remain in a healthy state.

Any impairment to the health of an organ affects the system to which it belongs; any impairment to a particular system affects other systems with which it works to keep you in good health.

"All parts of the body which have a function, if used in moderation and exercised in labours in which each is accustomed, become thereby healthy, well developed and age more slowly, but if unused they become liable to disease, defective in growth and age quickly."

— Hippocrates

1. The Skeletal System

We have all seen the model of the skeleton that hangs in the doctor's office. Or the stack of picture cards of the dancing skeleton that we used to carry around in our pockets. (Remember?)

The human skeletal system is the internal framework that supports the body (each human skeletal system has the same number of bones).

This system is composed of bone, connective tissue, cartilage, tendons and ligaments.

It holds your soft internal organs in place and protects them e.g. the skull protects the brain, the vertebral column protects the spinal cord, the rib cage protects the heart and lungs.

The skeleton also helps you to move – muscles are attached to the bones which give the muscles leverage to bring about movement through push and pull action. Flexibility of movement is aided by the presence of joints e.g. elbow joint, knee joint.

Bone also acts as a store for calcium (for bone strength) and bone marrow. Bone marrow aids in production of red blood cells so vital for the transfer of oxygen from the lungs to the cells.

2. The Respiratory System

The cells in the body require oxygen to stay alive. Short-term oxygen starvation causes brain damage; prolonged oxygen starvation leads to death.

Oxygen to sustain life is drawn into the body through the Respiratory System. Air intake flows along the system starting from:

the Nose and Nasal Cavity - → Mouth - → Pharynx - → Larynx - → Trachea - → Bronchi and Bronchioles - → Lungs - - → Alveoli

At the alveoli, oxygen is transferred to the cells; in exchange carbon dioxide and dissolved solid waste material from the cells are transferred to the blood (water content of the blood). Air exhalation then retraces the inward steps, leading the carbon dioxide to be exhaled to the outside world through the nose.

Another organ of the Respiratory System is the diaphragm. Located in the chest, the dome-shaped sheet of muscle separates the chest from the abdomen. When we inhale, the diaphragm is drawn downward, the muscles around the ribs pull them up making the chest cavity deeper and larger. This creates more air space. The more air we draw in, the more oxygen we get. The more oxygen in the body, the healthier we can be.

On exhalation, the diaphragm returns to its dome-shaped position. The shrinking of the air space forces air out through the nose.

In the nostrils, there is nose hair; then there is the mucous membrane that lines the passageway where the air passes through. The nose hair and the membrane serves to trap dust and other air impurities from reaching the lungs, keeping the air as clean as possible.

Not only does the Respiratory System work with the Muscular System to expand and contract the chest during inhalation and exhalation, it also works with the Circulatory System. Fresh, clean air is fundamental to our well-being.

3. The Circulatory System

The Circulatory System (also known as the Cardiovascular System) is centred on the heart which pumps blood in two circular loops:

- From the heart to the lungs and back and
- From the heart to the rest of the body and back.

Flow from the Heart to the Lungs and back:

Deoxygenated blood that is oxygen-depleted and containing carbon dioxide and metabolic waste products is brought back to the heart via the veins. This blood is pumped to the lungs to pick up oxygen, brought back to the heart before being pumped to the rest of the body.

This pulmonary flow to and from the lungs is as follows:

Veins (carrying d*eoxygenated blood from the body)* - - ->
Right side of Heart - - → Arteries (Pulmonary) - - →
Lungs (Alveoli) to pick up oxygen - - - >
Veins (Pulmonary)* - - -> **Left side of heart**
*Note that these are the only veins that contain oxygenated blood: all other veins contain deoxygenated blood

From the heart to the rest of the body and back.

The other circular flow of blood is from the Heart to and from the Rest of the Body. The heart pumps the blood which carries oxygen and nutrients to the cells in all parts of the body. The blood then transports the carbon dioxide to the lungs to be expelled. Other waste products are also transported from the cells to other organs like the liver and kidneys for processing and elimination from the body. The flow is:

Left side of heart - - > Arteries (oxygenated blood) - ->
Arterioles - - >
Capillaries (oxygen/carbon dioxide exchange) - ->

Venules - - > Veins - - > **Right side of Heart**

The constituent parts of blood are red blood cells, white blood cells, platelets, and liquid plasma. The blood that is being pumped round the body is a medium of transport for oxygen, carbon dioxide and other waste products. It also acts to protect the body (through its white blood cells) and regulates different aspects like the body's temperature.

Note the close working relationship between the Circulatory System and the Respiratory System. The Muscular System (cardiac muscles, blood vessels) is also involved, likewise the Digestive System for the transport of nutrients to all parts of the body after the food has been broken down in the stomach.

4. The Digestive System

This is the system that helps to digest the food you eat and the liquids that you drink. The digestive tract (also known as the alimentary canal or gastrointestinal tract) starts in your mouth (where food and drink enter), through the pharynx, down the oesophagus to your stomach, then through your intestines (both small and large) and finally ends at your anus through which we get rid of the solid waste produced by the body.

Food is chewed in the mouth, swallowed through the throat into the oesophagus leading to the stomach. In the stomach, the food is mixed with the stomach juices to break the food down even more before passing it to the small intestines for the nutrients to be absorbed into the blood stream. The indigestible parts of the food (dietary fibre) is then passed along to the large intestines to be defecated through the anus.

People used to say that "you are what you eat". It is more correct to say that *"you are what you eat and absorb"*. What you absorb depends to a great extent on the health of your digestive system. If the digestive system is not in good health, you can eat the most expensive foods in the world but the absorption rate will be low. You end up wasting your money on expensive food; most of the nutrients would end up exiting the body.

Know of skinny friends who eat like a horse but look like scarecrows? Chances are their digestive systems are not efficient in absorbing the nutrients.

Good nutritious food and a healthy digestive system go a long way to keep you in good health.

Do note the close working relationship between the Digestive and Circulatory Systems. Not only that, the Digestive System also works closely with the Skeletal and Muscular Systems – when you chew your food, when you swallow, when the oesophagus pushes the food down to the stomach through peristalsis, in the stomach when the food is churned and mixed with the gastric juices.

5. Muscular System

There are three types of muscles in the human body:

- skeletal (or striated) muscles which are voluntary in nature;
- cardiac muscles which are involuntary and
- smooth muscles which are also involuntary.

The skeletal muscles are the most obvious. We have all seen posters of muscular people. The muscles that they are so proudly displaying to us are the skeletal muscles – the muscles just under the skin. Skeletal muscles are used for movement. They can be controlled and commanded to carry out the tasks we want. That is why they are called "voluntary".

Smooth muscles (found in organs like the oesophagus, the stomach, the blood vessels and the bladder) are involuntary muscles which carry out their function without conscious control. When you swallow food or drink, the oesophagus will work automatically to transfer the material down to the stomach; the stomach automatically works to break down the food. You have no control over them. They just work by themselves.

Cardiac muscles (found in the heart and the walls of the aorta and the main vein) contract rhythmically and spontaneously without any human intervention. Cardiac muscles are also involuntary muscles. You have no control over the beating of your heart.

6. Nervous System

The brain and the spinal cord make up the Central Nervous System. The brain at the top is the hub of decision-making, the spinal cord (running down inside your backbone) is the main highway which serves to connect to the rest of the body.

Branching out from the spinal cord are numerous byways of neurons connecting to the various organs in the body. This network of nerves is the Peripheral Nervous System.

The nervous system is responsible for receiving, sending, and interpreting information from the external environment and helping the body respond in return. Messages are sent quickly and responses are usually short-lived.

The nervous system also monitors and coordinates internal organ function.

7. Sensory System

You have 5 senses – touch, sight, smell, taste and hearing. You feel touch through the skin, you see with your eyes, you smell with your nose, you taste with your tongue and you hear with your ears. Collectively, this is your Sensory System.

This system serves to bring information to the body, allowing it to receive, manage and respond to changes both within and outside the body.

You see danger, you move to avoid it. You feel raindrops, you know to get out of the rain. You taste bad food, you spit it out. You hear a commotion, you investigate. You smell freshly baked bread, you want some.

Your survival depends on these sense organs to alert the nervous system to help you survive.

8. Urinary System

The Urinary System is the body's filtering system. The main organs of the Urinary System are the two kidneys; they are supported by the two ureters, each connecting a kidney to the bladder which will hold the urine until it is time to go to the toilet. From the bladder runs the urethra through which the urine is passed out from the body. In the male, this is through the penis; in the female, it is through the urethral orifice.

Remember that a man's body is 60% water, a lady's is at least 50% water and a small child is greater than 60% water? Remember also that all three have to drink enough water throughout the day? What happens to all that water?

Healthy kidneys work really efficiently. As the blood (plus water, the body's metabolic wastes, toxins and foreign substances) is passed by the arteries through the kidneys, they filter these out, adjust the water level in the blood, and return the filtered blood to the veins leading out of the kidneys.

The urine produced is passed to the ureter, then to the bladder and finally exits the body through the urethra. Urine is 96% water and 4% dissolved metabolic waste. Of the water that you drink each day, 60% goes out of the body as urine; the other 40% goes out as sweat, faeces or through the lungs. The cleansed blood thus has the proper water level, the required salts and other materials.

The proper level of water in the blood keeps our blood pressure at the correct level. To maintain blood pressure at the proper level, three different body systems are working together - the kidneys (Urinary System) work together with the blood vessels (Circulatory System) and the spinal cord and brain (Nervous System) to adjust the water in the blood.

9. Endocrine System

In the human body, there are several glands that make up the endocrine system. The glands secrete hormones (chemical messages) which control various aspects of the body's functions. The hormones are released into the blood stream, taken all over the body and the target organ will pick up the message and take action – do something, refrain from something, or start something for another organ to detect.

These glands are, in alphabetical order, the adrenal glands, hypothalamus, ovaries, pancreas, parathyroid, pineal, pituitary, testes, thymus and thyroid. They work together to keep you healthy.

For example, the pancreas releases insulin to control the level of sugar in the blood. If the pancreas is not able to do its job, this can lead to diabetes. The pituitary gland is critical to growth, mental development and reproduction.

10. Lymphatic Immune System

The Lymphatic System is made up of the lymph ducts, lymph nodes, lymph vessels, lymph capillaries and the lymph fluid (containing proteins, electrolytes and white blood cells).

The role of the Lymphatic System is to defend the body against disease. Its job is to repel harmful bacteria, viruses and other foreign organisms from the body. If any of these gain entry into the body, the lymphatic system works hard to neutralise them. In the event that they still pose a danger to the body, the lymph cells will fight to kill the invaders.

The Lymphatic System works with the Muscular System to distribute the lymph fluid.

11. Integumentary System

When you look at a naked baby, what do you see? You see that the baby is covered by skin from the top of its head to the soles of the feet. Then there is the hair on the head; the finger nails at the tips of the fingers and the toe nails at the tips of the toes. This is the Integumentary System which serves to cover the body.

What does the skin do? It serves to protect your deeper tissues from physical damage, it keeps bad things out (germs and microbes), it helps to regulate the body's temperature and it helps the body to get rid of some metabolic body wastes. It also protects you from the sun.

Your Hair - is there any function apart from making you look good? Most definitely. Hair protects – eyebrows prevent sweat from going into the eyes, eyelashes protect the eyes, hair in the nostrils and outer ear trap foreign matter from entering.

Hair (your body hair) also does one more thing - keep you warm. Birds use their feathers to trap air to insulate their bodies against the cold air; beavers use their fur to do the same; you use your body hair to the same effect – trapping air, thus insulating the body from excessive heat loss.

What about your nails? Nails protect the tips of our fingers and toes. Innocuous but useful. Nails are also weapons for both aggression and self-defence. Notice the long nails that some people have?

12. Reproductive Systems

The twelfth system in the human body is dedicated to the preservation of our species. Without the ability to produce offspring, the human race will die out and become extinct. It is in our own interest to stay healthy to produce healthy offspring.

The human reproductive system has two parts – the male reproductive system and the female reproductive system. Reproduction is accomplished when the male and female come together with the purpose of having children.

In the man, the reproductive system is made up of the scrotum, the 2 testes (also known as testicles), the epididymis, a pair of spermatic cords, the seminal vesicles, the ejaculatory duct, the urethra, the prostate, the Cowper's glands, the penis and semen.

In the woman, the female reproductive system includes the ovaries, fallopian tubes, uterus, vagina, vulva, mammary glands and breasts.

For reproduction to take place, both the man and the woman have to be in reasonably good health for their reproductive systems to do their jobs.

Let us look at some examples of how your various body systems work together to take care of you.

Protection from the Environment

Imagine that you are freezing. How do the body systems react to protect you?

· Your skin (Integumentary System) feels (Sensory System) the cold. You are losing too much heat.
· The nerves (part of the Peripheral Nervous System) in your skin sends a message back to the spinal cord

(part of the Central Nervous System) saying "Very COLD"
· The signal goes to the brain (the decision maker in the Central Nervous System)
· The brain interprets the signal and decides that more warmth is needed.
· It sends a signal to the spinal cord – tell the skin muscles to trap more air.
· The signal goes to the muscles (Muscular System) to which are attached the follicles of the body hair.
· The muscle contracts to raise the hair to try and trap more air.
· Hence the goose pimples!

Protection from Injury

What happens when you accidentally brush your arm against a hot kettle?

· Your skin (Integumentary System) feels (Sensory System) the heat. It is very hot – "TOO HOT"
· The nerves (part of the Peripheral Nervous System) in your skin sends a message back to the spinal cord (part of the Central Nervous System) – "TOO HOT"
· The signal goes to the brain (the decision maker in the Central Nervous System)
· The brain interprets the signal and decides to move the arm away from the danger.
· It sends a signal to the spinal cord – tell the arm muscles (Muscular System) to pull the arm away to prevent further injury.
· The signal goes from the spinal cord to the nerves (another part of the Peripheral Nervous System) attached to the relevant muscles.
· The muscles contracts, leveraging on the arm bones (Skeletal System) to contract.

· This contraction of the muscles pulls the arm to safety.

Fighting Illness

What happens when you fall ill?

Your body's defences have been breached by its enemies - bacteria, viruses, toxins and other organisms. How did these get into the body? Basically, through the body's orifices – the nose through which we take in the air from the atmosphere, the mouth with which we eat and drink, the urethra with which we urinate, the anus with which we defecate, the genitals and breaks in the skin (scratches, scrapes, cuts).

Your body's defence mechanisms now go into battle to fight off these enemies. In this battle, if the defences hold, you will emerge relatively unscathed – weaker but not harmed to any great degree. The body will rebuild its immune system. If the defences break down, then you will be plunged into a more serious – even critical – situation.

Remember – the healthier you are, the easier it is to ward off illness.

> *"Take care of your body. It's the only place you have to live".*
>
> *- Jim Rohn*

Chapter 5

Getting Healthier: The Meaning

The Objectives

What is good health? What does "get healthier" mean? How is "health" measured? These are really good questions to which we need answers.

For the ordinary man in the street, good health is simply to:

- maintain an ideal weight,
- feel energetic all day long,
- have time to sleep for 7 to 8 hours each night
- have recreational time to do the things you love
- be relatively free of stress
- be free of medication as much as possible and
- have spiritual time to maintain our relationship with God.

The Factors Of Good Health

What does good physical health entail? Physical health is a combination of two factors – strength and endurance (fitness). Picture a scale - on one end of the scale is Poor Health and on the other end of the scale is Great Health. Good health sits in the middle of the scale.

```
Low Fitness            Good            Great Fitness
Poor - - - - - - - - - - - - - - - - - - | | - - - - - - - - - - - - - - - - - > Great
Low Strength           Good            Great Strength
```

Getting healthier is moving along the scale from the left end to the right end. It is a journey from a position of less strength and low fitness to a position of more strength and greater fitness.

33

Many of us have, inadvertently, slipped from the middle of the scale (good health) towards the left end of the scale (poor health). By doing nothing to take care of our health, it has deteriorated over time.

Many amongst us want to move in the other direction – back towards better fitness and greater strength. Getting healthier is a journey where a person, on any point of the scale, decides to embark on a journey to build up strength and to improve endurance. This effort to move to the right of the scale (or to stay exactly where you are after you have found your niche), is the essence of the journey.

The important point to remember is your present physical health is what it is today arising from your own set of circumstances. These are unique to you. Your health is what it is today because of things you did, or did not do, in the past. A person does not gain weight overnight; high blood pressure and diabetes also develop over time.

What matters most now is that you take stock of where you are today and where you want to be in the near future. Just as your less-than-satisfactory health condition built up over time, a more satisfactory health condition can be cultivated. All it needs is for you to take the steps that will help you move towards a healthier condition. It may be baby steps but as a famous quote goes, "The journey of a thousand miles starts with the first step".

> "The greatest thing in this world is not so much where we stand as in what direction we are moving."
>
> — von Goethe

The Current Situation

The point you are at, in simple terms, can be summed up as follows:

Current Diet + Current Lifestyle = Current State of Health

If you are unhealthy following this equation, carrying on in exactly the same way means that there is going to be no change; as you know, doing the same thing over and over and expecting different results is insanity.

What do you need to change? That is the question. If the current equation is not working, you need a new equation.

The good news is that there is a simple new equation that you can follow. The new equation to follow is:

Smarter Food Choices + Healthy Active Lifestyle = Better physical health

The two key areas that need re-examination are:

1. Food Choices (You are what you eat and what your body absorbs) and
2. Choice of Lifestyle (active lifestyle versus sedentary lifestyle)

By making simple changes in your daily diet and in your physical activity, you are going to discover a new you, one who is going to bring so much more joy and happiness to those around you.

The direction of the journey is clear – moving from a state of poor health to a better state of health. Methods can be followed; targets can be established; the timing can be estimated. All it needs is for you to commit to the change.

The Process

Note that getting healthier is a process. A person does not become healthy or unhealthy overnight but gradually over time.

Let me illustrate. Take a jug. Fill it with water to the brim.

- Add colour to the water – use food colouring, any colour will do.
- If you think that your health is average, add 3 drops of food colouring. If you are unwell, add 5 drops of the colouring.
- Stir the water to mix the colouring completely.
- The coloured water now represents your cells in your body.
- Now take a small cup and scoop out one cupful of water from the jug.
- Pour the water away. This represents your dead cells.
- Now fill the cup with clear water. This represents your younger, healthier cells assuming that you are taking better care of yourself.
- Pour this cup of clear water into the jug and mix well.
- The water in the jug is likely to be slightly less colourful than before.
- Repeat the process and the water should become clearer and clearer with each cupful. It represents you getting healthier over time.

Though we have used clean water in the above exercise, the water in the cup can be any one of three colours – clear (you become healthier) as shown above, same as the water in the jug (no change to your health) or of a deeper colour than the water in the jug (you are getting more unhealthy).

Understanding the above is critical. If you are not as healthy as can be, there is hope. Take better care of yourself and you can become healthier and healthier over a period of time.

Is there hope for people who are unwell to get better? YES!!! There is hope for all of us.

"The natural healing force within each of us is the greatest force in getting well."

— Hippocrates

Chapter 6

The Journey Model

Introduction

You would have heard this famous quote: "The journey of a thousand miles starts with the first step". Like most objectives, the first step is always the hardest. However, once the first step is taken, the ball will start rolling.

Getting healthier is exactly like going on a journey. Like any journey, there are 4 key factors that you need to know before starting out. In simple diagrammatic form, the representation of the 4 factors is as follows:

Starting Point is **A** -> **B** Destination (Your Goal)
                                      C How to Get from A to B
There is a fourth factor –   **D** Why? (the reason for the journey)

This model is really useful in that it can be used over and over again. Once a person reaches a goal, the model can be reset to take into account the new goal for starting a new journey.

The Key Factors

You have all driven on many journeys, taking road maps to guide you. Similarly, you have been on holidays, looking up Site Maps to guide you wherever you vacation.

Without fail, the first thing that you do is to find out your exact location. Once this is determined, you then check the other factors.

A. Where Are You?

The very first thing when you look at a road map or a site map is to find out exactly where you are. As the saying goes, 'X' marks the spot (You Are Here). *If you do not even know where you are to start with, you are well and truly LOST.*

B. Where Do You Want To Go?

Once you have figured out your starting point (you are no longer lost), the next activity is to look up your destination (where you want to be). This represents your goal. *If you do not know your goal, you will be clueless as to what to do next.* This reminds me of the 4 vultures in the Disney film "The Jungle Book". Four vultures – John, Paul, George and Ringo – are sitting on a branch. John asks the other three "what do you want to do?" Back comes the reply from them – "I don't know." Then Paul asks the other three - "what do you want to do?" The same reply comes back from John, George and Ringo – "I don't know." Then it is George's turn to ask - "what do you want to do?" John, Paul and Ringo shout back - "I don't know." Finally, it is Ringo's turn to ask the question. The same answer comes back – "I don't know."

Clarity of goal is important to success in a journey.

C. How Do You Want To Get There?

Having figured out both your starting point and your destination, you can now work out how to get from Point A to Point B. The "How" is your C. Can you walk? Do you drive? Should you take a train? Or fly? *Not knowing "How" means you are as good as stuck!*

D. Why?

Next comes the "Why". What is the purpose of this journey? The reasons can be many and varied. It can be as simple as

"I wish that I did not always feel so tired." Or "I want to look younger than I do". Maybe it is just "I wish I could keep up with my children and grandchildren". Or "I do not want to be the last person to be picked for team games".

Deep down, there is only one true reason. What is this one true reason for you? Find this out about yourself and this will be your motivation.

How do you know that you have hit the nail on the head? When you give this answer to the "why", you are likely to have teary eyes and go all emotional. That is when you know the true reason for your journey.

To sum things up, in any journey,
Not knowing A, your starting point, you are **lost.**
Not knowing B, your goal, you are **drifting**;
Not knowing C, how to get there, you are well and truly **stuck.**
Not knowing D, the reason for doing so, means you are **lacking commitment.**

Getting healthier is the same as going on a journey; you want to know all the 4 factors about the journey. You want to know about:

- **A** your starting point – so you **know where you are starting from**
- **B** your goal – this gives you **direction and focus**
- **C** your method – to give you **progress and hope**
- **D** your reason – to give you **purpose and commitment**

Your Starting Point

On any journey, there is packing to be done. You need to pack your essential stuff like toiletries, skincare, underclothes, night clothes, etc. Then there are things to pack for the occasion. If you are going to the beach, you pack your beachwear, your sunscreen lotion, etc. For a trip up the mountain, the clothes are entirely different.

In terms of getting healthier, it is no different. You need to take along some basic information (your luggage, so to speak). This information is to tell you where you are in terms of your health today - right now, right this minute.

What is your Point A in terms of your health?

To determine this, you need to know these 7 elements about yourself.

1. What is your height?
2. What is your present weight?
3. What is your Basal Metabolic Rate (BMR)? This is the amount of energy (calories) that your body burns when you are at rest.
4. What are your daily/weekly activities? Do you exercise? Are you taking part in any sporting activities? Or are you living a sedentary life?
5. What are your daily eating habits? What do you eat for breakfast, lunch and dinner? Do you snack in between, say at 11 am and 4 pm? What are these snacks? Do you take supper late at night? What do you take for supper?
6. Do you have any medical conditions that you need to factor in? Are you on medication for any medical ailments?
7. Do you indulge in any unhealthy habits like smoking, drinking alcohol, sleeping very late at night, taking late night suppers, etc.?

You need this basic information to help you determine the destination and the correct route to take, so to speak.

Initial Action

To find out how tall you are (element 1), a simple measuring tape will tell you.

A good body scanner can tell you how much you weigh and what your BMR is straight away (elements 2 and 3). A good scale to use is the popular Tanita scale, widely-used and sold world-wide.

As for activities and eating habits, you want to note down your daily activities and what you are eating for one week. This is input into the fourth and fifth elements.

As for element 6 (any medical consideration), factor this in. The route you take must take this into account. You must also let your medical practitioner and/or healthcare giver know what you plan to do in advance.

Always inform and consult your doctor and professional caregiver. They can provide vital input and help monitor your health status as you progress along the way.

As for the unhealthy habits (element 7), do list down your unhealthy habits. You know the common bad habits which harm you – smoking, drinking, not getting enough rest (e.g. staying up late to play computer games, online chats), etc. You want to stop these habits.

Your Reason Why

As for D (the reason for wanting to be healthier), you want to do a bit of soul searching. Motivation is all important in your efforts to be healthier and to stay healthier. Take the time to work this one out; things are not always what they appear to be. There is no right or wrong reason - just do your best to find out for yourself your true reason for undertaking this journey. This will keep you motivated as you go on this journey.

When you are motivated and committed, you will make every effort to reach your goals. You will be focussed and determined. Couple that with the most appropriate methods to reach your objective and you will really reap the rewards of your efforts.

Try this simple method to work out the true reason for your journey to better health. Take any reason you have and ask yourself WHY? To the answer, ask WHY once more. Keep on asking why to each succeeding answer until you cannot answer WHY any more. This is likely to yield your reason for the journey to better health.

How do you know when you have the right answer? The right answer will make you go all teary-eyed; it will give you goose pimples.

The Journey Starts

Let me state from the beginning that this is a journey to learn about how to take better care of your health. Be assured that this is going to be a really interesting journey.

At the beginning of a journey, any journey, you need to know the following:

a. Starting Position
b. The direction to take and
c. The Final Destination (Goals)

At this point in time, the "How" to get there is not yet decided.

Starting Position – Health Statistics

As mentioned previously, you need the following details even before setting off.

- your height,
- present weight,
- body fat %,
- visceral fat reading,
- Basal Metabolic Rate (BMR),
- daily/weekly activities,
- daily food intake,
- medical ailments/medication and
- habits which are harming us health-wise.

With the above information, you can establish your starting point (Point A). As yet, you still do not know your destination (your goal – Point B). Remember the four vultures in the movie "The Jungle Book"? Not knowing where to go, you also cannot formulate any action plan to get there (Point C).

So, what is your goal? How do you use the information that you have gathered so far to help you decide the direction that you should take and the final destination so that you know when you have reached your goal.

Setting The Direction

To determine your new general direction, make use of the information that you have gathered about your height, your weight and body fat %. Using your height, you can quickly calculate what your *"ideal weight range"* should be.

Let us calculate the recommended weight for any given height using the formula below.

For men
(Your Height in centimetres) less (100 cm for men) = our Ideal Weight in kilograms
Ideal Weight in kilograms less 5 = lower indicator of Ideal Weight Range
Ideal Weight in kilograms plus 5 = upper indicator of Ideal Weight Range.

For Ladies
(Your Height in centimetres) less (110 cm for ladies) = our
Ideal Weight in kilograms
Ideal Weight in kilograms less 5 = lower indicator of Ideal
Weight Range
Ideal Weight in kilograms plus 5 = upper indicator of Ideal
Weight Range.

You can then compare this range with your present weight to give you your present status.

You are overweight if your current weight is greater than the Ideal Weight Range; you are underweight if your current weight is less than the Ideal Weight Range; or you are within the calculated Ideal Weight Range. This gives you a clear indication of the **direction** that you should head:

- *lose body fat* (if you are overweight) or
- *put on lean muscle* (if you are underweight) or
- *maintain weight* (if you are within the stipulated range), although you may have to shape up a bit.

Using the indicators derived from your personal information, you know the general direction to follow. This is critical.

Setting The Overall Goal

Getting the direction correct is important. Lose body fat? Go South. Gain muscle mass? Go North. Maintain weight or reshape our body composition? Go East or maybe even West. It means you now have an idea of where to go.

You now have your own personal road map showing you the direction. But you also need to know "by how much???" How do you know this? This is where you have to do some simple arithmetic once again. You all know the saying "the devil is in the details."

Setting The Objectives

Weight Management

If you are in the *lose body fat group*, the calculation is:

Your Present Weight *less* the top range of Your Ideal Weight. The positive number gives you an indication of the Kilograms in body fat you have to lose.

If you are in the *gain muscle mass group*, the calculation is the same:

Your Present Weight *less* the top range of Your Ideal Weight. The negative number gives you an indication of the Kilograms in lean muscle mass (NOT body fat) you have to gain.

If you are in the *maintain weight group*, you are lucky. But you may still have some work to do, depending on your body fat % reading. You may have more body fat and not enough muscle mass!

What Weight Should We Aim For?

Using the hard facts above, aim for the mid-to-top of the range for the weight factor. Many a time those aiming for the mid-to-bottom of the range end up looking skinny and gaunt.

Body Fat Composition

For all three groups, there is a table to guide you on what your ideal body fat % should be, given your age and gender (whether male or female).

The table for **men** is as follows:

Body Fat Index for Men

Age	Excellent	Healthy	Medium	Obese
20 – 24	10.8	14.9	19.0	>23.3
25 – 29	12.8	16.5	20.3	>24.3
30 – 34	14.5	18.0	21.5	>25.2
35 – 39	16.1	19.3	22.6	>26.1
40 – 44	17.5	20.5	23.6	>26.9
45 – 49	18.6	21.5	24.5	>27.6
50 – 54	19.2	22.1	25.1	>28.2
55 – 59	19.8	22.7	25.6	>28.7
60+	20.2	23.3	26.2	>29.3

The table for **Ladies** is as follows:

Body Fat Index for Ladies

Age	Excellent	Healthy	Medium	Obese
20 – 24	18.2	22.1	25.0	>29.6
25 – 29	18.9	22.0	25.4	>29.8
30 – 34	19.7	22.7	26.4	>30.5
35 – 39	21.1	24.0	27.7	>31.5
40 – 44	22.6	25.6	29.3	>32.8
45 – 49	24.3	27.3	30.9	>34.1
50 – 54	25.2	28.2	31.8	>35.1
55 – 59	26.6	29.7	33.1	>36.2
60+	27.4	30.7	34.0	>37.3

You want your body fat % to be in the "Excellent" or "Healthy" band.

You now have two very clear road signs to guide you – how many kilograms to lose or gain, and what % of body fat to lose or gain as well.

Everyone needs some body fat. So long as you are in the "Excellent" or "Healthy" band, you are in good shape.

Visceral Fat Danger

There is one crucial health reading you need to understand. This is the visceral fat content inside you. What is visceral fat? Simply put, it is fat that surrounds your vital organs in the trunk/ stomach area.

When you slaughter a chicken and cut it into two halves, you can see that there is fat in the chicken. One type of fat is that under the chicken's skin; this fat is all over the body. This is the body fat. You also have body fat under your skin.

When you look at the chicken's innards, you also see some fat surrounding the chicken's vital organs – the heart, lungs, etc. This is the visceral fat. When you do not take good care of yourself, you end up with high visceral fat. This is usually manifested in a man's "beer belly" and "love handles"; but make no mistake about it, even a skinny man can have a high visceral fat deposit. This "miserable fat" increases the risk of many ailments – high blood pressure, heart disease, bad cholesterol and diabetes (in its various stages).

Do not think that visceral fat is harmless. Visceral fat is not just a lump of inert fat. It is doing much to make you feel unhealthy. For a start, those with high visceral fat usually have big beer bellies. They are generally short of breath most of the time. This is because the fat in the abdomen is pushing up against the lungs, squishing them. The result – the lungs cannot expand to their full capacity, causing breathlessness.

The visceral fat is also pressing against the kidneys which in turn would scream for more blood. The result – blood pressure goes up.

Food that has gone bad is full of toxins; if you eat bad food, chances are you will get food poisoning. Visceral fat is like food that has gone bad sitting inside you. It is releasing toxins into your blood every day, slowly poisoning you. It is no wonder that people with high visceral fat feel unwell most of the time.

The liver has to work extra hard to clean up the toxins released each day. This leads the liver to get agitated; there is no rest for it. An agitated liver produces bad cholesterol in you.

Breathlessness, higher blood pressure, toxins and bad cholesterol. All this from a lump of fat deep inside you. Take action today to get rid of the beer belly and love handles as quickly as you can in a simple and safe way.

What is a good level of visceral fat that you should aim for? The chart says:

1 – 4: Good (ideal)   5 – 8: Healthy (still all right)
9 – 12: Bad   Over 13: Alarming

Take care to be in the 1 - 4 band; at worst, you should be in the 5 – 8 band, no higher. Any reading above 8 is not good; any reading above 12 is a medical disaster waiting to happen.

Compared to body fat, the effort and commitment needed to get rid of visceral fat is much more. But it will be worth it to feel healthy again.

Personal Baggage

When you travel, you usually take along some "personal baggage". What is this personal baggage? It is not the physical type of baggage but your personal habits – eating, drinking, recreational, resting, and sleeping. Take stock of these habits, critically examine them in some detail and decide what to get rid of and what new, healthier habits to cultivate.

You need to check the following habits about yourself:

- Do you take regular meals or do you take meals as and when you like?
- Do you starve yourself and then go on a binge when you are hungry?
- Do you feel hungry often? Do you constantly crave for food?
- Do you habitually eat fast foods, instant foods or processed foods?
- Do you drink a lot of sugary drinks like colas, etc?
- Do you drink alcohol regularly?
- How much water do you drink a day?

Take stock of your eating habits and record them in a table like the one shown here.

Current Eating Habits

Meal	Time	What I Am Eating
Breakfast		
Mid-morn		
Lunch		
Mid-afternoon		
Dinner		

Current Activity Habits

What are your present activity habits and how have you been feeling recently?

- Are you active or are you a couch potato?
- How often do you exercise each week (if you do exercise at all?)
- Do you get tired easily?

- Do you feel unwell or fall sick often?
- Do you suffer from chronic headaches or migraine, backaches, constipation?
- Do you feel stressed at the office? At home?
- Are you smoking heavily?
- Are you getting enough sleep each night?

Knowledge about the daily activities is important as you want to adjust the BMR to take these activities into account to establish your Total Metabolic Rate (TMR) for the day. This fact will help in meal planning.

Chapter 7

Food Philosophy and Diet

Introduction

There are six different food groups that you need to sustain your health:

- Carbohydrates
- Proteins
- Fats
- Fibre
- Vitamins
- Minerals

Each food group is best suited for its designated principal function.

Produce in the Carbohydrates group are good for producing energy; those in the Protein group are good for their amino acids (for muscle building). But they are by no means mutually exclusive. A food source for protein would also contain some Carbohydrates and Fats; within the Fibre group, a produce would also contain amounts of both Vitamins and Minerals. A produce in any one food group can also supply the nutrients of another food group.

You just need to know which to eat more of, which to eat less of and which to avoid if you can. And, overall, you need to know how much to eat in a given day.

Food Philosophy

A key choice to make upfront about food and nutrition concerns three little words. Arranged in one order, it leads you to better health; arranged in the reverse order, it leads to more health challenges.

What are these three words that can impact you so much? They are:

o *Eat to Live or*
o *Live to Eat*

The first philosophy means an approach of moderation, eating when you are hungry to take care of yourself, not overindulging; taking pleasure in the foods you love and yet not subjecting your body to the vagaries of gluttony. Eating sensibly yet not denying yourself the pleasures of good food.

The second philosophy is the direct opposite of the first, eating what pleases you regardless of whether you are hungry or not. In this group, thoughts are always on food and on what to eat; indulgence without thought as to the necessity of it. Eating for the sheer pleasure of eating, whether the food is good for you or otherwise.

If your present philosophy is the first, please continue on this track; if it is the latter, I can only urge you to rethink. This simple change in perception affects all your action regarding your approach to your health.

Remember this quotation:

> "Let food be thy medicine and medicine be thy food."
>
> — <u>Hippocrates</u>

Diet

Eating the right foods is important; also just as important are how much you eat and how well you balance the calories you take in with those you burn off.

Basically:

The Right Food + Right Quantity + A Little Physical Activity = Healthy You

> "If we could give every individual the right amount of nourishment and exercise, not too little and not too much, we would have found the safest way to health."
>
> — Hippocrates

You are conversant with overdoing something and neglecting something else that is also as important. A simple example is a bodybuilder who concentrates on exercises for the upper body but neglects the lower body. What is the result? A bodybuilder who looks great from the waist up but with spindly legs from the waist down! Notice the imbalance?

True health is based on balance, not extremes. Follow a balanced diet; your food is enough to give you most of the nutrition you need. There should be minimal need for taking supplements. The first step, therefore, is to make sure that your meals are well balanced and nutritious.

It is also important to understand that the nutrients supplied by a particular food group also need the nutrients from other food groups for better absorption and utilisation of your food. That is why your plate of food should be balanced - divided into 4 parts of 25% each of Carbohydrates, Proteins, Fibre and Fruits.

Chapter 8

Carbohydrates

Introduction

What is the function of carbohydrates? **Carbohydrates** is the food group that gives you energy for all the activities of the day. Carbohydrates are the best source of energy for the body.

When you consume carbohydrates, your digestive system will convert them into glucose for your cells. Glucose is the only type of sugar that the human body can burn to produce energy. All cells need glucose to function – for the brain to think, for the muscles to move, for the heart to beat. No glucose equals no energy.

Carbohydrates can be divided into two categories – simple carbohydrates and complex carbohydrates. Let us look at an analogy.

Let's Go Camping

What do you do when you go camping?

One important activity is to collect wood – fuel for the camp fire. You search for various types of wood – twigs and thin sticks, slightly thicker branches, well-dried and ready for starting a fire; yet even thicker branches, a little bit damp maybe but still good for burning for when the fire is burning steadily.

You use the twigs and thin sticks to start the fire; the twigs catch fire fast, but the flames are small and short-lived.

Once there is a steady flame going, you add the slightly thicker, dry pieces to make the flame bigger, steadier and longer-lasting. You keep adding similar pieces of wood till there is a steady, blazing fire. You use this to boil water, cook food, keep warm and light your camp.

On the periphery of the fire, you put the thicker, maybe slightly damp, pieces of wood. The heat from the fire will dry out the wood. Once all the chores are done and everyone is ready to retire for the night, you put the thickest pieces of wood into the fire.

These pieces will burn slowly and steadily through the night. In the morning, there are the glowing ambers from which you can rebuild the fire.

Other bigger pieces of wood that are too damp and too big cannot be used as firewood. Burning these will create smoke and soot and cause the fire to die out.

The key points to take from the analogy are:

- The different types of wood needed for the fire.
- The difference in the flammability of the wood.
- The unsuitability of some of the wood for burning.

A Simple Comparison

When Building A Fire

Wood - - - - - > Burn - - - - - > Fire - - - - - > Energy - - - - - > Activities (cook, boil, light . .)
(twigs, etc)

Food - - - - > Digest - - - - > Sugars - - -> Energy - - - - - > Activities (walk, run, warm . .)
(carbohydrates)

When Eating

Now let us see the key points between wood and carbohydrates in their respective functions.

Key Points

Fire		**Food**
Wood	1	Carbohydrates
- different Types		- Simple; Complex
Flammability	2	Glycaemic Index
- how easy to burn		- Low, Medium, High
Type of Flame	3	Type of Sugars
- Suitability for Purpose		- Glucose, Glycogen, etc

There are two types of carbohydrates – simple and complex. Simple carbohydrates are the twigs and sticks that are used to start the fire. Complex carbohydrates are the thicker branches, slower burning, longer lasting and giving more heat.

In food terms, the glycaemic index indicates how fast a food item is converted into sugar in the human body.

The higher the figure, the faster that food item is converted into sugar. Generally, simple carbohydrates have a high glycaemic reading and complex carbohydrates have a lower reading. The food item with the lower number has less impact on the sugar level in the blood in the short term.

Then there is the glycaemic load to consider. This is the quantity of the food item consumed multiplied by its glycaemic reading to give the glycaemic load. For example:

100 grams of Food A x Glycaemic Reading of 100 = 10000 (Glycaemic Load).

100 grams of Food B x Glycaemic Reading of 50 = 5000 (Glycaemic Load).

Other things being equal, it is better to choose Food B because its glycaemic load is lower.

Simple carbohydrates come in large part from sources like corn meal, potatoes, short grain white rice, instant white rice, glutinous rice, cereals, pasta, bread and some fruit and vegetables (legumes). Complex Carbohydrates would be from items like brown rice, spaghetti, sweet potato, yams.

No matter where you live, you have good choices. The simple rules are:

- to buy local;
- buy seasonal;
- favour low glycaemic foods over high glycaemic foods.

Over the long term, low glycaemic foods are better for your health. High glycaemic foods contain sugars that burn very fast and give you an immediate energy surge. However, you get hungry faster and will yearn for more of the same. Low glycaemic foods, on the other hand, burn more slowly, keeping you full for a longer period of time. Here are some staple foods sorted by their glycaemic readings.

Staples

Low GI	Medium GI	High GI
Barley - Pearled		
Beans - Black		
Beans - Garbanzo		
Beans - Kidney		
Beans - Lima		
Beans - navy		
Beans - Pinto		
Buckwheat		
Fettuccini - Egg	Corn	
Lentils	Cornmeal	

Noodles - Instant	Couscous	
Pasta - Wheat Shapes	Gnocchi	
Peas - Dried	Millet	
Potatoes - New	Potatoes - Baked	Potatoes - French Fries
Potatoes - Sweet	Potatoes - Canned	Potatoes - Fresh Mashed
Ravioli - Meat		Potatoes - Instant Mashed
Rice - Brown	Rice - Basmati	Rice - Glutinous
Rice - White long grain	Rice - Chinese Vermicelli	Rice - Instant White
Spaghetti	Rice - Wild	Rice - Short Grain White
Tortellini (Cheese)	Taco Shells	Tapioca
Wheat tortilla		
Yam		

Whatever staple food you are currently consuming, there are alternatives. Do your best to switch to another staple with a lower glycaemic value.

I am sure that in the short list above, you will be able to find the types of staple food that you love; I am also positive that there is enough variety in the list to give you variety in your meal plans so that you do not get weary of eating the same stuff day after day.

Good food does not have to be expensive and boring; you can shop smartly and your meals can taste great at the same time.

Chapter 9

Proteins

Introduction

The cell is the basic building block of life. It is made up of protein. Proteins consist of building blocks called amino acids and there are more than 20 different types of amino acids. Of these, there are 8 which are called essential amino acids. Essential amino acids are so named because the body cannot make them; these must be provided in the food you eat (just like essential fatty acids). The human body can make the rest of the other non-essential amino acids from these 8. The eight essential amino acids are Isoleucine, Leucine, Lysine, Methionine, Phenylalanine, Threonine, Tryptophan, and Valine.

There are two classes of proteins – complete and incomplete. To qualify as a "complete" protein, the 8 essential amino acids must be present in the food source in roughly equal quantity.

The function of proteins is to help the body grow and repair itself. Protein makes up about 12% of the total weight of the body, regardless of gender. Adult men need about 50 – 60 grams of protein per day; adult ladies need 40 – 50 grams per day. Insufficient protein intake can cause decreased Immunity, stunt growth and can also cause heart and respiratory failure.

Complete proteins are generally derived from animal meats (chicken, beef, turkey, lamb). Animal meats will provide not only protein but animal fats, minerals and vitamins as well (refer to table below).

Source	Protein	Fat	Minerals	Vitamins
Beef	Yes	Yes	Magnesium Phosphorus Potassium Sodium Iron Selenium Zinc	B12 D K
Chicken	Yes	Yes	Potassium Selenium Zinc	B12 D
Lamb	Yes	Yes	Iron Selenium Zinc	B12 K
Pork	Yes	Yes	Potassium Sodium Selenium Zinc	B12
Turkey	Yes	Yes	Phosphorus Potassium Sodium Copper Iron Selenium Zinc	B12 D E K
Veal	Yes	Yes	Potassium Copper Manganese Selenium Zinc	B12

When taking animal meats for their protein, do choose the lean cuts instead of the cuts which are marbled with fat. This will keep your consumption of animal fats to a minimum.

Seafood is also a very good source of protein – cod, salmon, sardines, shrimp, tuna, scallops or whatever is plentiful and economical in your area. In addition, seafood provides plenty of vitamins and minerals.

Source	Protein	Omega3	Minerals	Vitamins
Anchovies	Yes	Yes	Sodium	D
				K
Cod	Yes	Yes	Magnesium	D
				C
Herring	Yes	Yes	Magnesium	B12
			Phosphorus	Magnesium
			Potassium	E
			Sodium	
Sardines	Yes	Yes	Calcium	B12
			Magnesium	D
			Phosphorus	E
			Potassium	
			Sodium	
			Chloride	
Caviar	Yes	Yes	Calcium	B12
			Magnesium	D
			Sodium	
Catfish	Yes	Yes	Potassium	B12
Perch	Yes	Yes	Calcium	B12
			Magnesium	
			Phosphorus	
			Potassium	
Pollock	Yes	Yes	Calcium	B12
			Magnesium	
			Phosphorus	
			Potassium	
			Sodium	
Salmon	Yes	Yes	Magnesium	B12

			Phosphorus	
			Potassium	
Tuna	Yes	Yes	Magnesium	B12
			Phosphorus	
			Potassium	

Do try to eat fish at least twice a week. Given a choice of all the proteins, choose fish for one simple reason – you get the Omega 3 fatty acids which are not available from animal meats. The more "oily" fish (salmon, tuna, mackerel, sardines) pack a fair amount of essential fatty acids (omega 3) which is good for your health. So you are getting double the benefit in this source of protein.

Dairy products like milk, cheese, yogurt and eggs are also good sources of complete proteins. Eggs are a really good source for complete protein (6 grams of protein in one egg) and are easy to prepare e.g. boiled eggs. Other good sources are:

* cheddar cheese
* goat's cheese
* whole cow's milk
* goat's milk
* eggs (boiled)

For vegetarians who cannot have access to vegetables with complete proteins, there is no cause for concern – just take a mix of different vegetables with each meal to get all the essential amino acids you need. What is missing in one food choice can be supplemented by another with the required amino acid. Just like a jig saw puzzle – put the pieces together to get the whole.

For those who choose not to consume animal or dairy products, complete proteins can also be obtained from some grains and nuts. Amongst these would be quinoa, buckwheat, hempseed, chia, soy, rice and beans (in combination).

The eight essential amino acids for adults are Phenylalanine, Valine, Tryptophan, Threonine, Isoleucine, Methionine, Leucine and Lysine. Use this list to help you evaluate protein drinks if you need protein supplementation. Make sure all 8 are present in roughly equal amounts in your selected supplement.

Chapter 10

Fats and Oils

Introduction

The average fat content in the human body is between 15 to 22%, influenced by what you eat, how you exercise, your age (it generally increases with age but not necessarily so), gender (male 15; female 22), and your genetic disposition.

Fats and oils are an essential part of a healthy diet. It is incorrect to think that we must avoid taking them totally. The fact is that you need some fat – but the right kind of fat. There are good fats, bad fats and really bad fats. You just have to make sure that you take only the good fats and avoid the bad fats.

Unsaturated fats are the healthy fats; saturated and trans fats are the unhealthy ones. In the first group are produce such as olive oil, avocados, almonds, flaxseed, fatty fish (like salmon, sardines and tuna). Produce in the second group are meats with high fat content, fried foods, packaged snacks.

Do your best to take Omega 3 fatty acids daily; these are important for your health. The three Omega 3 fatty acids are ALA (alpha-linoleic acid), DHA (docosahexaenoic acid) and EPA (eicosapentaenoic acid). Of the three, ALA is an essential fat i.e. it cannot be manufactured by the body. It must be consumed in the diet. AHA is found in plant sources like nuts and grains (for example, chia seeds, flaxseed, quinoa, soy beans and walnuts) and vegetables like Brussel sprouts and cauliflower.

The other two crucial ones – EPA AND DHA – can be made by the body from ALA but in very limited quantities. Therefore we need to eat foods that are rich in DHA and EPA, foods like fish and shellfish, especially the "oily" fish like salmon, mackerel, sardines, rainbow trout, shrimp, tuna and herring. That is why a healthy diet should include at least two portions of fish a week. Fish that is steamed, baked or grilled is a healthier choice than fried fish.

Depending on your diet preferences, the information below should help you to identify the sources of the three Omega 3 fatty acids. For those who are strictly vegetarians or vegans, you need to eat more vegetables, grains, nuts and seeds to get more ALA for the body to convert into DHA and EPA.

Sources of ALA

From vegetables – soybeans, Seaweed, spirulina, leeks, Navy beans, Pinto beans, kale, broccoli, cauliflower, lettuce (butterhead), lettuce (red leaf), spinach.

From nuts and seeds – flaxseed, butternuts, walnuts, chia seeds, walnuts, beechnuts, soybean, hickory nuts, pecans, almonds, peanuts.

From fruits – avocados, raspberries, strawberries.

From Grains – oats germs, wheat germ, barley bran, rice bran, wheat bran.

From Legumes – soybeans, common beans, cowpeas, lima beans, garden peas, chickpeas, lentils.

Sources of EPA and DHA

From Fish – Salmon, herring mackerel, anchovy, sardines, trout, shark, sword fish, sea bass, Pollock, Whiting, flounder, sole, halibut, carp, mullet, tuna; perch; snapper, haddock, eel, catfish, cod, pike

From seafood – mussel; spiny lobster; oyster; crab; shrimp; octopus; clam; scallops; conch.

Chapter 11

Fibre

Introduction

Vegetables are really good for your health; in vegetables, you will find nutrients and fibre.

Fibre (also called dietary fibre) is a complex carbohydrate and are of two classes - soluble or insoluble. Soluble fibre is of the type that can be broken down by the digestive system and provides energy. Insoluble fibre (also known as roughage) cannot be broken down by our digestive system, and does not provide energy.

Soluble fibre is found in many vegetables including green leafy vegetables, celery, carrots and many others. In the case of carbohydrates, the important consideration is the glycaemic index; for dietary fibre, the colour of the vegetable is the important factor. The different colours indicate the presence of different nutrients. The main idea is to select vegetables of different colours for a meal so that you get a mix of different nutrients.

Colour Groups: Vegetables

Brown/ White	Green	Red	Yellow/ Orange	Blue/ Purple
Non-Starchy				
Cauliflower	Asparagus	Radicchio	Cantaloupe	Eggplant
Garlic	Broccoli	Radishes	Carrots	Purple asparagus
Ginger	Brussel Sprouts	Red bell peppers		Purple cabbage
Mushrooms	Celery	Red chili		Purple carrots
Onions	Cucumbers	Red onions		Purple peppers
Shallots	Green Pepper	Rhubarb		
Turnips	Leafy Greens	Tomatoes		
	Leeks			
	Lettuce			
	Okra			
	Spinach			
	Watercress			

Brown/ White	Green	Red	Yellow/ Orange	Blue/ Purple
Starchy				
Parsnips		Red potatoes	Butternut	
Potatoes		Kidney beans	squash	

Brown/White	Green	Red	Yellow/Orange	Blue/Purple
Tapioca White corn			Pumpkin Sweet corn Yellow potatoes Yellow winter squash	

For most people, the staple food is already starchy; it is better to complement that starchy staple with lots of leafy greens and fruits instead of more starchy vegetables.

Soluble fibre is also found in many fruits.

Colour Groups: Fruits

Brown/White	Green	Red	Yellow/Orange	Blue/Purple
Bananas	Green Apples	Cherries	Apricots	Blackberries
Brown pears	Green grapes	Raspberries	Grapefruit	Blueberries
Figs	Limes	Red apples	Lemons	Plums
Dates	Kiwifruit	Red grapes	Mangoes	Prunes
White peaches		Strawberries	Nectarines	
		Watermelon	Oranges	
			Papayas	
			Peaches	
			Pineapples	
			Rock melon	
			Sultanas	

Why is there this emphasis on making sure that there are colourful vegetables and fruits on our plates? Having a mix of colours on your plate means that you are getting different nutrients in your diet.

At each meal during a week, do eat vegetables and fruits from different colour groups (at least two to three) on different days of the week.

Health Benefits in the Colour Groups of Vegetables and Fruits

Properties	Brown/ White	Green	Red	Orange/ Yellow	Purple/ Blue
Anti-viral	Yes				
Anti-bacterial	Yes				
Potassium	Yes				
Anti-cancer		Yes	Yes		Yes
Folate		Yes			
Healthy Heart			Yes		Yes
Healthy Eyes		Yes	Yes		
Healthy Mucous Membrane				Yes	
Anti-Cataracts				Yes	
Anti-Stroke					Yes
Cell Protection					Yes
Improves Memory					Yes
Healthy Ageing					Yes

Insoluble fibre is that part of the vegetables and fruits that you eat which cannot be broken down in the digestive system. It serves two purposes:

- it makes you feel full and
- it also helps clean out the digestive tract as it makes its way through to the large intestines.

The more fibre you take, the faster it is that food moves through your digestive system. This reduces the time that the indigestible part of the food that you take stays in your digestive tract, especially in the colon.

Imagine leaving uneaten food in a bowl out in the open. Overnight, the food starts to decay. If you attempt to eat this food, your body will reject the food by making you throw up. Your body is rejecting all the toxins present in the decaying food.

The colon holds all the faecal matter before you pass it out from the body when you move your bowels. This faecal matter is full of toxins. Your body becomes unhealthier the longer you let faecal matter stay in your body. So the more fibre you eat, the faster you get rid of the unwanted faecal matter from your system.

This is one of the reasons why you want your plate of food to be at least 50% vegetables and fruits, apart from all the vitamins and minerals that you get from them.

Chapter 12

Vitamins

Introduction

In the food that you eat, there are nutrients which your body needs in relatively small quantities but which play essential roles in regulating your health. These micronutrients (so called because of the small quantities required of each) cannot be manufactured by the body; you must get them from the food you eat.

When you eat the other food groups like carbohydrates, protein, fats and fibre (macronutrients), these are broken down further by the body. For micronutrients, however, the body uses them whole, without further breaking them down.

One group of micronutrients is called Vitamins (the other is Minerals). Vitamins are organic food substances found only in living things, i.e. plants and animals. They are essential for your body to function properly, to promote growth, to give energy and for your general well-being. With very few exceptions the human body cannot manufacture or synthesize vitamins. These must be supplied in our diet or in man-made dietary supplements.

Remember the campfire analogy? Think of vitamins (together with minerals) as the flints that provide the sparks that start the fire.

There are 13 such vitamins, divided into two groups:
- a fat soluble group (vitamins A, D, E and K) and
- a water soluble group (vitamins B1, B2, B3, B5, B6, B7, B9, B12 and C).

Fat soluble vitamins can be stored in the body for later use when needed; water soluble vitamins will be passed out from the body through the urine.

Way back in the era of sailing ships, voyages took months. In the conditions on board, fresh vegetables and fresh fruits spoilt quickly. Sailors and all on board were therefore deprived of the micronutrients to be found in fresh fruits and vegetables. The lack of Vitamin C over a protracted period of time led to sailors developing scurvy – manifested by bleeding gums and lethargy. Similarly, a prolonged lack of vitamin D caused rickets, a condition marked by soft, weak bones that can lead to skeletal deformities such as bow legs.

In poor economies in today's environment, prolonged Vitamin A deficiency can cause blindness.

Here are some more examples of the value of vitamins to your health.

The fat soluble vitamin A (retinol) prevents night blindness, helps recovery from colds and bursitis (inflammation) between bones and muscles. It also improves eyesight. Do you want healthy hair, skin, teeth and gums, and healthy mucous membranes? Make sure your diet contains vitamin A; it helps.

Vitamin D (calciferol) works to prevent colds and helps the body in utilising calcium and phosphorous. Vitamin D also helps in assimilating vitamin A.

Vitamin E (Tocopherol) helps to prevent heart and blood disorders. It helps improve fertility and normal production. It also helps in utilising vitamin A.

Vitamin K (Phylloquinone) helps your liver to function properly and promotes proper blood clotting.

Many decades ago, the recommended daily intake of the respective vitamins were governed by what is called the RDA (Recommended Daily Allowance). This RDA was the quantity needed to stave off particular illnesses. Modern research recommends the ODA (Optimum Daily Allowance). The new higher quantity serves to protect the body, not just to stave off illness.

The table below shows the older RDA and the newer ODA.

Vitamin	Name	Recommended Daily Allowance (RDA)	Optimum Daily Allowance (ODA)
Fat	**Soluble Vitamins**		
A	Retinol	800 mcg	2500 mcg
D	Calciferol	5 mcg	30 mcg
E	Tocopherol	10 mg	250 mg
K	Phylloquinone	80 mcg	80 mcg
Water	**Soluble Vitamins**		
B1	Thiamin	1.2 mg	35 mg
B2	Riboflavin	1.7 mg	35 mg
B3	Niacin	20 mg	100 mg
B5	Pantothenic acid	7 mg	200 - 400
B6	Pyridoxine	2 mg	25 mg
B7	Biotin	0.3	
B9	Folic Acid	0.4	
B12	Cobalamin	1 mcg	25 mcg
C	Ascorbic Acid	60 mg	2000 mg

The above table can serve as a guide for you to buy vitamin supplements (if necessary). Do make sure that the required vitamins are on the nutrition label and that the quantity per serving (or per tablet/ capsule) is more than the RDA and closer to the ODA.

Sources of Vitamins

From fruits – in descending order of completeness of providing vitamins B, excluding B12. Vitamin B12 is the one vitamin that is available only from fish, poultry, meat or dairy sources in food.

Vitamin B Series -   From Fruits

B1	B2	B3	B5	B6	B9
Avocado	Avocado	Avocado	Avocado	Avocado	Avocado
Cherimoya	Cherimoya	Cherimoya	Cherimoya	Cherimoya	Cherimoya
Dates	Dates	Dates	Dates	Dates	Dates
Breadfruit		Breadfruit	Breadfruit	Breadfruit	Breadfruit
Guava		Guava	Guava	Guava	Guava
Mango	Mango	Mango		Mango	Mango
Pomegranate	Pomegranate		Pomegranate	Pomegranate	Pomegranate
	Lychee	Lychee		Lychee	Lychee
	Passion Fruit	Passion Fruit		Passion Fruit	Passion fruit
Boysenberries		Boysenberries			Boysenberries
Grapes	Grapes			Grapes	
Loganberries		Loganberries			Loganberries
Pineapple				Pineapple	Pineapple
Watermelon			Watermelon	Watermelon	
	Banana			Banana	
			Gooseberries	Gooseberries	
Grapefruit			Grapefruit		
Orange					Orange
			Raspberries		Raspberries

Black Currants   Blackberries

Mulberries   Nectarine

Prickly Pear   Peach   Papaya

Starfruit   Strawberries

From vegetables – in descending order of completeness of providing vitamins B, excluding B12.

Vitamin B Series -	From vegetables				
B1	B2	B3	B5	B6	B9
Spirulina	Spirulina	Spirulina	Spirulina	Spirulina	Spirulina
Brussels Sprouts	Brussels Sprouts		Brussels Sprouts	Brussels Sprouts	Brussels Sprouts
Okra		Okra	Okra	Okra	Okra
Peas	Peas	Peas		Peas	Peas
Potatoes		Potatoes	Potatoes	Potatoes	Potatoes
	Squash - winter	Squash - winter	Squash - winter	Squash - winter	Squash - winter
Sweet Potato	Sweet Potato	Sweet Potato	Sweet Potato	Sweet Potato	
Butternut Squash		Butternut Squash	Butternut Squash	Butternut Squash	
Corn		Corn	Corn	Corn	
French Beans	French Beans		French Beans		French Beans
Lima Beans	Lima Beans			Lima Beans	Lima Beans
Parsnips		Parsnip	Parsnip		Parsnip
	Amaranth Leaves			Amaranth Leaves	Amaranth Leaves
	Artichoke	Artichoke			Artichoke
Asparagus	Asparagus				Asparagus
	Bok Choy			Bok Choy	Bok Choy
			Broccoli	Broccoli	Broccoli
	Mushrooms	Mushrooms	Mushrooms		
	Pumpkin	Pumpkin	Pumpkin		
		Spaghetti Squash	Spaghetti Squash	Spaghetti Squash	

Chinese Broccoli			Chinese Broccoli
	Squash - summer		Squash - summer
			Beetroot
		Celeriac	Chinese Cabbage
		French Beans	
		Green Pepper	
		Kale	
Swiss Chard		Taro	Spinach

Vitamin B Series -   **From Nuts and Grains**

B1	B2	B3	B5	B6	B9
Rye	Rye	Rye	Rye	Rye	Rye
Wheat - Durum	Wheat - Durum	Wheat - Durum	Wheat - Durum	Wheat - Durum	Wheat - Durum
Wheat - Hard Red	Wheat - Hard Red	Wheat - Hard Red	Wheat - Hard Red	Wheat - Hard Red	Wheat - Hard Red
Wheat - Hard White	Wheat - Hard White	Wheat - Hard White	Wheat - Hard White	Wheat - Hard White	Wheat - Hard White
Buckwheat	Buckwheat	Buckwheat	Buckwheat		Buckwheat
Chestnuts	Chestnuts		Chestnuts	Chestnuts	Chestnuts
Oats	Oats		Oats		Oats
		Sunflower Seeds	Sunflower Seeds	Sunflower Seeds	Sunflower Seeds
Filberts/ Hazelnuts				Filberts/ Hazelnuts	Filberts/ Hazelnuts
Peanuts		Peanuts			Peanuts
Quinoa	Quinoa				Quinoa
Rice Brown				Rice Brown	

Spelt   Spelt

Pistachios   Pistachios

Brazil Nuts   Almonds   Barley

Cashews

Flax Seed

Macadamia Nuts

Millet

Pumpkin Seeds

Pecans

Pine Nuts/Pignolias   Walnuts

| Vitamin B Series - | Legume Sources | | | | |
B1	B2	B3	B5	B6	B9
	Edamame	Edamame	Edamame	Edamame	Edamame
	Soy Beans	Soy Beans	Soy Beans	Soy Beans	Soy Beans
Black Eye Peas			Black Eye Peas	Black Eye Peas	Black Eye Peas
	Adzuki Beans	Adzuki Beans	Adzuki Beans		
Navy Beans	Navy Beans			Navy Beans	
Winged Beans	Winged Beans	Winged Beans			
	Fava Beans	Fava Beans			
	Garbanzo Beans			Garbanzo Beans	
Kidney Beans				Kidney Beans	
			Lima Beans	Lima Beans	
	Mung Beans		Mung Beans		
	Pinto Beans			Pinto Beans	
		Split Peas	Split Peas		
White Beans				White Beans	
Black Beans		Pigeon Beans			

Vitamins B12 and D from All Sources

	B12	D
Meat	Beef	Beef
	Beef Sausage	Beef Sausage
	Beef Hot Dog	Beef Hot Dog
		Bacon
	Chicken (Ground)	Chicken Breast
	Lamb	
	Pork	
		Turkey Bacon
		Turkey Hot Dog
		Turkey Ground)
	Veal	
Dairy	Cheddar Cheese	Cheddar Cheese
	Cow's Milk	Cow's Milk
	Eggs	Eggs
	Yogurt	Yogurt
	Cottage Cheese	
		Cream Cheese
		Goat Cheese
		Sour Cream
		Whipping Cream
	Lowfat Yogurt	
Seafood	Caviar	Caviar
	Cod	Cod
	Hamburger	Hamburger
	Herring	Herring
	Sardines	Sardines

Anchovies

Catfish

Perch

Pollock

Salmon

Tuna

The good part about eating fish for protein is that it also provides the healthy fats, especially Omega 3 fatty acids, for your body.

Chapter 13

Minerals

Introduction

Minerals are elements that originate in the soil and cannot be created by living things, such as plants and animals. Yet plants, animals and humans need minerals in order to be healthy. Plants absorb minerals from the soil, and animals get their minerals from the plants or other animals they eat. Most of the minerals in the human diet come directly from plants, such as fruits and vegetables, or indirectly from animal sources. Minerals may also be present in your drinking water, but this depends on where you live, and what kind of water you drink (bottled, tap). Minerals from plant sources may also vary from place to place, because the mineral content of the soil varies according to the location in which the plant was grown.

You can get the minerals you need from the plants, fish, animals and fluids you ingest.

Sources of the major Minerals

From Fruits

Calcium	Magnesium	Phosphorus	Potassium	Sodium	Chloride
Blackcurrants	Blackcurrants	Blackcurrants	Blackcurrants		
Dates	Dates	Dates	Dates		
	Passion Fruit	Passion fruit	Passion fruit	Passion Fruit	
Pomegranate	Pomegranate	Pomegranate	Pomegranate		
	Avocado	Avocado	Avocado		
	Breadfruit	Breadfruit	Breadfruit		
	Guava	Guava	Guava		
	Kiwi	Kiwi	Kiwi		
Mulberries	Mulberries	Mulberries			
Prickly Pears	Prickly Pear		Prickly pear		
	Banana		Bananas		
Blackberries	Blackberries				
	Cherimoya		Cherimoya		
Grapefruit			Grapefruit		
		Lychee	Lychee		
	Watermelon		Watermelon		
Orange	Loganberries		Cherries		
	Raspberries		Chinese pear		
			Papaya		

From Vegetables

Calcium	Magnesium	Phosphorus	Potassium	Sodium	Chloride
Amaranth leaves	Amaranth leaves	Amaranth leaves	Amaranth leaves	Amaranth leaves	
Spirulina	Spirulina	Spirulina	Spirulina	Spirulina	

French Beans	French Beans	French Beans	French Beans		
Swiss Chard	Swiss Chard		Swiss Chard	Swiss Chard	
	Artichoke	Artichoke		Artichoke	
Bok Choy			Bok Choy	Bok Choy	
Brussels Sprouts		Brussels Sprouts		Brussels Sprouts	
Butternut squash	Butternut squash		Butternut squash		
Celery				Celery	Celery
	Lima Beans	Lima Beans	Lima Beans		
Parsnip		Parsnip	Parsnips		
		Celeriac		Celeriac	
Kale				Kale	
Okra	Okra				
	Peas	Peas			
		Potatoes	Potatoes		
		Pumpkin	Pumpkin		
			Sweet Potatoes	Sweet Potatoes	
			Bamboo Shoots	Beetroot	
Chinese Broccoli		Corn		Broccoli	
				Fennel	Lettuce
					Olives
					Rye
				Spaghetti squash	Seaweed
Turnip		Taro			Tomatoes

From Nuts and Grains

Calcium	Magnesium	Phosphorus	Potassium	Sodium	Chloride
	Pumpkin Seeds	Pumpkin Seeds	Pumpkin Seeds	Pumpkin Seeds	
Oats	Oats	Oats	Oats		
Wheat - Durum	Wheat - Durum	Wheat - Durum	Wheat - Durum		
Wheat - Hard	Wheat - Hard	Wheat - Hard	Wheat - Hard		
White	White	White	White		
Amaranth	Amaranth			Amaranth	
	Buckwheat	Buckwheat	Buckwheat		
Brazil Nuts	Brazil Nuts	Brazil Nuts			
	Quinoa	Quinoa		Quinoa	
	Rye	Rye	Rye		
	Wheat - Hard Red	Wheat - Hard Red	Wheat - Hard Red		
	Almonds		Almonds		
	Cashews	Cashews			
			Coconut	Coconut	
	Pine Nuts/ Pignolias	Pine Nuts/ Pignolias			
Pistachios			Pistachios		
		Spelt		Spelt	
		Sunflower Seeds	Sunflower Seeds		
Filberts/ Hazelnuts	Peanuts			Chestnuts	
Sesame Seeds					

From Meats

Calcium	Magnesium	Phosphorus	Potassium	Sodium	Chloride
	Beef	Beef	Beef	Beef	
		Turkey Bacon	Turkey Bacon	Turkey Bacon	
			Pork Sausage	Pork Sausage	
			Ground Chicken	Bacon	
			Pork	Beef Sausage	
			Veal	Beef Jerky	
				Beef Hot Dog	
				Turkey (Ground)	
				Turkey Hot Dog	

From Dairy

Calcium	Magnesium	Phosphorus	Potassium	Sodium	Chloride
Cheese - Cheddar	Cheese - Cheddar	Cheese - Cheddar		Cheese - Cheddar	Cheese - Cheddar
Goat Milk	Goat Milk	Goat Milk	Goat Milk	Goat Milk	
Yogurt (Low Fat)	Yogurt (Low Fat)	Yogurt (Low Fat)	Yogurt (Low Fat)	Yogurt (Low Fat)	
Cheese - Goat		Cheese - Goat		Cheese - Goat	
Cows Milk			Cows Milk	Cows Milk	
Yogurt			Yogurt	Yogurt	
Cottage Cheese				Cottage Cheese	
Cream Cheese				Cream Cheese	
Eggs				Eggs	
	Soy Milk			Soy Milk	
Sour Cream					

From Seafood

Calcium	Magnesium	Phosphorus	Potassium	Sodium	Chloride
Sardines	Sardines	Sardines	Sardines	Sardines	Sardines
Pollock	Pollock	Pollock	Pollock	Pollock	
	Herring	Herring	Herring	Herring	
Perch	Perch	Perch	Perch		
Caviar	Caviar			Caviar	
	Salmon	Salmon	Salmon		
	Tuna	Tuna	Tuna		
	Cod		Catfish	Anchovies	

From Legumes

Calcium	Magnesium	Phosphorus	Potassium	Sodium	Chloride
Edamame	Edamame	Edamame	Edamame		
Soy Beans	Soy Beans	Soy Beans	Soy Beans		
White Beans	White Beans	White Beans	White Beans		
Winged Beans	Winged Beans	Winged Beans		Winged Beans	
	Adzuki Beans	Adzuki Beans	Adzuki Beans		
	Pinto Beans	Pinto Beans	Pinto Beans		
Navy Beans	Navy Beans	Navy Beans			
	Black Beans	Black Beans			
	Black Eye Peas	Black Eye Peas			
		Kidney Beans	Kidney Beans		
		Lima Beans	Lima Beans		
		Fava Beans			
		Garbanzo Beans			
		Pigeon Beans			

There are many more minerals and trace minerals (those which are needed by the body in really small quantities). Examples are chromium, copper, iodine, iron, etc. If you eat plenty of colourful vegetables and fruits, you should get enough of these.

Chapter 14

Balance

Introduction

Modern research reveals that a vitamin or mineral does not work in isolation but in combination with other vitamins, minerals and nutrients. For example, taking calcium, vitamin D, vitamin K, magnesium and phosphorus keeps bones strong and protects them against fractures. The fluoride helps bone formation as well as prevent dental cavities from starting or getting worse.

Here are some more examples of the co-operative work done by the various nutrients from the different food groups.

Vitamins A and K, and the minerals chromium, copper, iodine, iron, manganese, zinc, boron, nickel, vanadium and molybdenum are needed for your overall well-being.

To help burn carbohydrates for energy, these vitamins are needed - thiamine, riboflavin, niacin, b6, folate (folic acid), B12, pantothenic acid, biotin and choline.

Strong bones and teeth require calcium. For proper absorption of calcium, the body also needs other minerals like magnesium and phosphorus plus Vitamin D.

A healthy immune system needs the antioxidants vitamins C and E, the mineral selenium, and beta carotene found in vegetables and fruits in the red, orange and yellow groups. Vitamin A helps convert the beta carotene into vitamin A when you are exposed to sunlight.

For heart health and mental alertness, the fatty acids ALA, EPA and DHA are required plus a satisfactory supply of nutrients. Insufficiency of vitamin B3, vitamin B6, vitamin C, and the minerals zinc and magnesium negates the Omega 3 fatty acids that you consume.

Chapter 15

Physical Activity

Introduction

Who was Hippocrates? Hippocrates was a Greek physician who lived more than 2500 years ago. He is popularly referred to in Western culture as the "father of modern medicine." Some of his quotes, made during his lifetime, are just as relevant today as back in his time. One such quote is:

> *"That which is used - develops. That which is not used wastes away."*
>
> — *Hippocrates*

From the earliest days, physical prowess was critical to human survival. Humans hunted and foraged for food, relying on wits and physical ability to survive. *The human body was, and is, built for physical activity.* Inactivity actually results in a faster deterioration of the body's capabilities.

In the modern age, physical activity has been reduced to the two-thumb type. Can you guess what it is? You are right – two thumbs working feverishly on a smart device!

Let's Get Physical

It is so easy to keep your physical capabilities in reasonably good working condition with some simple physical activity three times a week, 30 minutes each time, totalling only 90 minutes per week. Just go for a walk.

"Walking is man's best medicine."

— Hippocrates

Put on your cleanest dirty clothes! Jeans, t-shirt, socks and a pair of walking shoes will do. After all, your objective is to get sweaty. After the walk, the clothes can go straight into the laundry.

Have some water with you when you go for your walk. It is important to stay hydrated as you exercise.

Before any exercise, it is important to loosen up so as not to injure any body part. Remember what the PE (Physical Education) teacher taught you in your younger days? Remember those warming up exercises? Do those exercises for 5 minutes first, loosening up your body from the neck, shoulders, arms, hips, legs and ankles.

Now you are ready.

- Start by standing in an area of your house where you are not in anyone's way.
- You are relaxed; your muscles are relaxed; your breathing is normal.
- Put your right hand on your left chest; feel the beating of your heart. The rhythm slow and easy.
- Your breathing is also shallow and slow.
- Your skin is dry i.e. you are not sweating.
- You are feeling your normal self.
- Now start to walk on the spot – raise your knees higher than normal as you walk. Jog slowly on the spot if you can.
- Keep walking (or jogging) for the next 5 minutes. Stop if you start to feel breathless before the five minutes are up.
- At the end of 5 minutes, stop.
- Now feel your heart; it is beating faster.

- You are breathing more heavily
- Your skin feels wet – with sweat.
- You may feel a little unsteady if you have not exercised for a long time.

Now you need to cool down first by doing some stretching exercises.

- Take a small sip of water.
- Perform stretching exercises.
- Upon completion, rehydrate by taking more water.

The stretching exercises help keep the aches and pains in your body to a minimum by removing the lactic acid in the muscles.

Your Achievement

What has this simple 5-minute walk done for you?

a. The Skeletal and Muscular Systems

Using the skeletal system as leverage, your muscles enable you to move. If you do not use your muscles, they atrophy (grow smaller and weaker). Simple exercises keep your muscles strong and toned. Older folks have a tendency to fall and Injure themselves because their muscles are weaker and can't help them to maintain their posture and keep their balance.

b. The Respiratory System

Over the course of your 5-minute walk, notice how your breathing goes from slow and shallow to fast and deep. As you engage in walking, your body starts to burn energy. It now requires more oxygen to keep up the activity. So the Respiratory System responds. Each breath you take is known as its vital capacity; the deeper the breath, the greater is the vital capacity.

The greater the vital capacity, the more efficient the oxygen/ carbon dioxide exchange in the lungs. More oxygen to the cells means more nutrients for the cells with each breath.

Within a given time, more frequent deep breaths means greater ventilation of the lungs (more air taken in for a given length of time). Like a room with many windows, opening just one window means that less fresh air comes in and less stale air is flushed out. Opening more windows leads to a greater inflow of fresh air and a faster removal of stale air. Deeper breaths is the equivalent of opening more windows.

As you exercise, the other parts of the body (e.g. the muscles, the brain) require more oxygen. The Respiratory System works faster to get oxygen to the lungs as quickly as possible. The chest muscles open up rib cage even more so that the lungs have more room to expand. This results in more air intake to the lungs per breath.

There have been studies that the lack of oxygen in the body leads to diseases; learning how to get more oxygen into the body keeps you healthy.

c. The Circulatory System

The Circulatory System comprises the heart, the blood vessels (the arteries and the veins) and the blood. With exercise, the heart pumps harder and faster to drive the blood through the arteries, firstly to the lungs (to pick up oxygen) and then to the rest of the body, especially to the muscles where the exertion is taking place. The faster flow of oxygenated blood results in more oxygen and nutrients for the exercising muscles.

To accommodate the faster beating of the heart, the arteries also dilate to carry more blood to the cells.

At the cells, the oxygen in the red blood cells is exchanged for the carbon dioxide and other waste materials produced by the other cells. The venous blood containing the carbon dioxide is transported to the lungs to be exhaled; other metabolic waste material is transported to the liver and kidneys for processing and disposal.

The exertion also causes the veins to transport the blood back to the heart much faster than before.

How do you know that the exchange of oxygen and carbon dioxide has taken place? Blood in the arteries is bright red, depicting its rich oxygen content. Blood in the veins is a dull red, showing its lack of oxygen and high carbon dioxide content.

The brain has to do one more thing also – to redirect blood from where it is not needed to where it is most needed. So it sends signals to body organs to do so. A good example will be blood flow to the stomach. Since you are not eating, blood is not needed in the stomach for digestive activities. Blood in the stomach is reduced and more blood is sent to the muscles being exerted.

(Now I know why Mum used to tell me – "do not run around when you have just eaten" or "do not take a bath immediately after your meals". She would make us wait 30 minutes before allowing us to do either after a meal. After meals, the stomach needs the blood more than your muscles.)

d. The Integumentary System

The body is constantly producing sweat as a way to regulate the body's temperature. In hot weather, you sweat more to keep the body cool; in cooler weather, you sweat less.

With exercise, more energy is used up and the body heats up more than usual. It needs to be cooled to maintain your body temperature at the correct reading.

Exercise also produces more waste material for removal from the body. To cool the body and remove the waste, the skin starts to sweat.

e. The Nervous System

Meanwhile, the Nervous System (both the Central Nervous System and the Periphery Nervous System) also works hard. It receives, interprets and acts in quick succession to keep up with your body's movements. It directs the chest muscles to open the rib cage more than before for greater air intake; it redirects more blood to flow to the muscles that are working; it regulates your body's temperature by generating sweat.

The increased physical activity also induces the brain and the nervous system to produce endorphins – hormones which help you to feel more alert. You must have heard people say "I feel so refreshed" after exercise and washing up. This is the work of the endorphins.

f. The Immune System

Physical activity over time leads you to a higher level of fitness. The fitter you are, the stronger is your immune system. You fall sick less often. And when you do, recovery is much faster.

g. The Reproductive System

It is no secret that the fitter you are, the greater the chances of producing offspring.

Your Enjoyment: Doing What You Love

You derive many benefits by including some simple exercise into your daily routine. This simple exercise can be any one, or all, of the activities that you loved in our childhood.

Remember the simple and fun activities that you used to take part in – walking, jogging, skipping (jump rope), playing catch, playing ball, doing the hula hoop, tossing the Frisbee with friends and family, doing the twist, or the Zumba, and many, many others like these. It does not matter what activity you choose. Just pick the physical activity that you love. The key point is to be active, not sedentary.

If you work and/or live in a high-rise building, try using the stairs for part of the way each time you go up or go down. Get off a few floors before your destined get-off point and use the stairs for the rest of the way. You will be surprised how much healthier you will become in a short space of time. Once you are fitter, you can increase the use of the stairs to get even fitter.

Or you can go to the park and walk. Take your family members with you. Bond with your family. Help them to get healthier.

Make new friends at the park. Breathe in the fresh air. Feel the warmth of the sun. Enjoy the beauty all around you.

As Frank Kafka said – *"Anyone who keeps the ability to see beauty never grows old."*

Chapter 16

Rest and Recreation

Introduction

From the moment you wake up in the morning till you go to sleep at night, your spring gets wound tighter and tighter throughout the course of the day. It is no wonder that you feel irritable at the end of the day – you are so wound up! Your blood pressure has probably gone up without your knowledge. You want to release this pressure during the day itself.

Just Breathe

To unwind, take short breaks during the day to focus on your breathing.

Your breathing is normally very shallow. You are not using your lung capacity and you are, therefore, getting less oxygen for your body. *Breathe more deeply* to get more oxygen for your body. The result can be amazing.

Do this simple experiment. Check out the colourful items around you. Note down how you feel. Now close your eyes. Put the tip of your tongue against the back of your top front teeth. Inhale as deeply as you can through your nose. Then exhale forcefully through your mouth. Do this for three minutes. Now open your eyes. Feeling more relaxed? Thoughts are more positive?

Colours are more vibrant? You achieved these changes simply through getting more oxygen into your body by breathing deeply.

Breathing technique for relaxation – find a quiet corner during a break in your routine. Sit upright and relax. Now close your eyes. Put the tip of your tongue against the back of your top front teeth. Clear your mind. Breathe in through your nose to the count of 8; hold your breath to the count of 4, breathe out through your mouth to the count of 8, hold your breath to the count 4. Repeat for as long as you wish.

Notice how relaxed you feel after this short exercise? Do this simple exercise two to three times a day to de-stress.

Increasing Your Lung Capacity

Breathe in deeply through your nose. Feel your stomach expand first, then your rib cage. Now exhale forcefully through your mouth. Suck your navel in towards your spine as you exhale. Do this for up to twenty times at least two to three times daily e.g. in the mornings, in the afternoons and at night. Feel the difference that it makes? There is one other benefit – you will get a flatter stomach over time if you practise this regularly.

Sleep

The human body - a living, breathing collection of cells and organ systems - is used to a daily cycle of light (day) and darkness (night). The day is a time for activity; night is a time of rest and sleep. It is when you sleep that all your internal organs work hard to carry out their respective maintenance routines. Each organ has its own housekeeping schedule at a different time of the night.

On average, an adult needs at least 7 – 8 hours of sleep each night. This sleep is best taken between 10 pm at night till 6 am in the morning to facilitate all the maintenance routines by the various organs.

There are many on-going studies on sleep, its benefits, the health challenges posed by lack of sleep and sleep deprivation. Examples of the health challenges are mental alertness, obesity, blood pressure, heart functions, ageing.

To minimise the risk of falling victim to these health challenges, you must do your best to get your 7 – 8 hours of restful sleep each night. Give your body a chance to repair itself. Get sufficient sleep each night.

A good laugh and a long sleep are the best cures in the doctor's book.

Irish Proverb

Chapter 17

Pluck These Low Lying Fruits

Please note that these health tips are for a person of normal health who is not under medical advice of any sort. Please check with your doctor or health care giver first to make sure that it is all right for you).

Introduction

There are many simple changes that you can make today to get healthier. Here are some of these which can be implemented quickly, safely and economically.

Start Today
Drink More Water

Water is the source of life. Water is essential for the chemical reactions that sustain life. Water makes up about 50% of the total body weight of a female; for men, the figure is 60%. (In a new born baby, the figure is as high as 80%).

Daily, you use water to wash clothes, clean dishes, take a shower, mop floors, etc. You make sure that you use enough water to ensure that things are clean.

You clean yourself externally daily, but you rarely think about cleaning yourself internally. Yet your internal body, especially your digestive system, needs cleaning just as badly, if not more so. Every day, you eat and you drink; and what goes inside your body? Besides the food, you ingest oil, chemicals, preservatives, hormones, insecticides.

How can you help the body to get rid of all these? Through water – through your urine, bowel movements, and sweat. If you do not drink enough water, you cannot clean your insides sufficiently.

How much water should you drink each day to stay hydrated? (Water means drinking water, not coffee, tea, colas, and the ilk.) As a general rule of thumb, a man needs to drink at least 3 litres of water a day; a lady needs to drink at least 2.2 litres of water a day.

To be more accurate,

For a man: Weight (in kgs) x 0.6 e.g. 70 kgs x .6 = 4.2 litres per day

For a lady: Weight (in kgs) x 0.5 e.g. 70 kgs x .5 = 3.5 litres per day

Start on the road to better health straight away, as early as tomorrow.

If you already have a water bottle, use the bottle that you have.

- If you do not have one, buy yourself a good water bottle (a 1 litre or 2 litre bottle will do).
- Buy a lemon (NOT lime) from the market or supermarket.
- On the night before you start this little exercise, make a note of how you have been feeling. Are you feeling tired most of the time? Are you low on energy? Do you have frequent headaches? Are you constipated? Just jot down your ailments.

On the morning of the day that you are starting this habit:

1. In the morning, fill your water bottle to capacity with drinking water.
2. Cut three thin slices out of that lemon, retaining the rind. (Keep the rest of the lemon for the next day).

3. Put the three thin slices of lemon, rind and all, into your water bottle. Do not squeeze the lemon for its juice; just put the slices straight into the water whole).
4. Drink that water throughout the day whenever you feel thirsty. Better still, set your watch or smartphone to alert you every hour on the hour. Drink at least 300 ml every time you get the alert. Over 10 hours of your waking day, you will finish 3 litres.
5. When you run out of water during the day, just add more water to the lemon slices in your bottle and drink that water.
6. At the end of the day, wash out your water bottle, throwing away the lemon slices.
7. On the morning of the next day, repeat the process from step 1 to 6.

At the end of one week, evaluate how you feel. Compare how you are feeling now after one week of drinking water with the lemon slices in it. Do you feel less tired now? Are you more energetic than at the start of this experiment? Are your headaches less frequent or totally gone? Are you a bit more regular in moving your bowels?

You will notice some physical differences within one week. These are likely to be positive.

Start the practice today!

If you like the results after one week, do share this tip with your family and friends.

Breakfast is the Most Important Meal of the Day

Many people today skip breakfast or have a quick breakfast (toast, fruit juice and coffee). Some call a coffee that they grab on the way to work "breakfast". The common thing about these "breakfasts" is that there is little or no nutrition in them. Some carbohydrate, sugar, low fat, but no protein.

Try taking a protein drink for breakfast. Why?

You have just woken up from sleep. Practically, you have been fasting over the last number of hours – no food and no drink whilst sleeping. Your cells are hungry and thirsty. They are ready to eat. Absorption is going to be at the highest level. The protein drink will be absorbed in next to no time.

Protein drinks are fast to make. Put the required number of scoops in a shaker cup. Add the requisite amount of water. Shake it up well to dissolve the protein powder. Drink it and you are set for the morning.

Breakfast is also the best time for food with low sugar content. Your blood sugar will not spike up and your pancreas need not be called into action to secrete insulin to bring the blood sugar level down to acceptable levels.

This home breakfast is less expensive than the coffee you pick up on the way to work. So much more nutritious too.

A Healthy Lunch to Keep You Awake

For the office workers and those providing other non-manual services, lunch can be very tempting. The usual practice is to have a nice lunch; after lunch it is normal to feel sleepy.

The lunch that you normally take is one with lots of carbohydrates, a little bit of vegetables and some protein.

The better alternative is a plate that is:

- 50% Vegetables and Fruit of various colours
- 25% lean protein
- 25% carbohydrates (preferably complex carbohydrates like brown rice, quinoa – not short-grained white rice).

To make sure that your lunch is a healthy one,

- load your plate with leafy greens and raw or grilled vegetables.
- add some protein —grilled chicken, beef or lamb (of the lean kind), fish, boiled eggs. (Eat more fish if you can).
- leave room for the fruits and plain water (not the colas and the like).

Take as little carbohydrates as possible during lunch; it is this that makes you sleepy in the afternoons.

To prove this point to yourself, for your next lunch, do not take any carbohydrates at all. Just take protein, vegetables, fruits and plain water. Then monitor how your afternoon goes compared to those afternoons when you had your normal lunch. Do not be surprised to find that you are more alert, energetic and productive compared to those afternoons when you had lots of carbohydrates during lunch.

Eat carbohydrates in moderation. 25% of your plate – not more.

Never eat till you are full

Following on, the key principle is to not eat until you feel really full. When you are about 80% full, stop eating.

Never starve yourself

On the opposite end of the scale, never starve yourself. If you are in a sedentary job, when you starve yourself or eat irregularly, the lack of food and physical activity makes the body think that there is a crisis. No food plus no activity equals crisis. Your body does not know when the next meal will come.

So when you take your next meal, the body will hoard the food sugar, keeping it for the hard times it thinks is coming. This will lead to fat build-up, contrary to logic. You think no food leads to weight loss; in fact, starving yourself and eating irregularly leads to weight gain!

So, never starve yourself. Take small, healthy meals regularly.

Avoid late night suppers

Some people like to take late night suppers. Some people like to eat all hours of the day and night. Now there are more 24-hour eateries than ever.

When you eat late at night then go to sleep, the stomach has not had time to digest the food. It stays in the stomach for much longer than it should. There is a common saying that goes "all diseases start in the stomach". Faecal matter that stays in the colon poisons us slowly; undigested food that stays in the stomach does the same.

Avoid late night suppers.

All Purpose Healthy Snack

Snack on hard boiled eggs.

Boil a few eggs at a time and keep the extras in the refrigerator.

Add some cherry tomatoes and some lettuce leaves to your hard boiled eggs.

Drizzle of olive oil or Italian Dressing; add salt and pepper.

This healthy snack will assuage your hunger and give you more protein. One egg gives you 6 grams of protein. (Adult men need about 50 – 60 grams of protein per day; adult ladies need 40 – 50 grams per day).

This can also be a good breakfast. Prepare this the night before and keep it in the fridge. You can then eat it the next morning, have your drink then go straight to work. More protein, better health and more savings.

Chapter 18

Be Grateful

Make Each Day A Great Day

Physically, you have to address issues of food, physical activity, fresh air and sunshine in your quest to be healthier. On the emotional level, you also want each day to be great. You want to face all that the day has in store with equanimity.

These are some simple ways to enrich each day on the emotional level.

Start Your Day Right

Every morning, before all and sundry rush out the door to go their separate ways,

* Give each of your loved ones in your household a 30-second hug.
* This should be a really close hug - chest to chest.
* Hold each loved one tight - like there is no tomorrow.
* Just close your eyes and enjoy each of them for at least 30 seconds

Your day will start that much brighter. You will not believe the love and affection that this simple hug will generate. The hugs you give are nothing compared to what you will receive in return.

Many of my friends and their families have found, to their surprise, the positive changes that they have experienced just because they started out each day as outlined above.

I would be very pleased to hear from you the results you are getting from this early morning routine.

Recharge Yourself During The Day

In the course of your day's activities, there will be things happening that may please you; there will be others that displease you or irritate you. Your spring will be wound up.

Do not forget to breathe. During the mid-morning and mid-afternoon breaks (or even during your lunch break),

* Find a quiet corner where you will not be disturbed.
* Sit down in an upright position – no sprawling.
* Close your eyes
* Put the tip of the underside of your tongue against the back of your top front teeth
* Now focus on your breathing
* Breathe in through your nose to the count of eight
* Hold your breath to the count of four
* Now breathe put through your mouth to the count of eight
* Hold your breath to the count of four
* Repeat this 8x4x8x4 breathing for as many minutes as you can
* Concentrate on the rhythm of your breathing all the while – no other thoughts

When you are finished doing this, you should be refreshed, ready to go again.

That inner spring that has been winding itself during the day has unwound itself a little bit just because of the few minutes you took to recharge yourself.

End Your Night Right

From the moment you wake up till you go to bed each night, you will receive many blessings. It is good that you acknowledge your blessings for the day. Express your gratitude.

Every evening, as you lie in bed before nodding off:

* Give thanks for all the good things that you have received this day – say them out softly to yourself as you lie in bed.

* List as many blessings as you can – from the big things to the little things. You will be surprised at how long this list can be.

* When you have finished expressing your gratitude for what you have received for the day, take the time to ask for what you would like to receive the next day – more of the same? Something really special? Just ask.

* On completion of this, you are ready for bed.

This expression of gratitude can bring so much inner peace and contentment into your life.

In Parting

My Wish For You

1 Have Faith in Yourself - believe that you can be healthier still
2 Recognise the Potential that is yours to be healthier
3 Take the Action to fulfil that Potential
4 Get the Results that you strive for

He who has health, has hope; and he who has hope, has everything.
Arabian Proverb

Wishing you Great Success

References and Further Reading

Human Physiology
1. Man's Body – An Owner's Manual
2. Woman's Body – An Owner's Manual
3. The Illustrated Atlas Of The Human Body by Beverly McMillan
4. http://www.innerbody.com

Cellular Nutrition
1. http://www.whfoods.com/nutrientstoc.php

Food Groups and Nutrition
1. Fats that Heal, Fats That Kill by Udo Erasmus
2. http://www.medic8.com/healthguide/articles/foodgroups.html
3. https://www.consumerlab.com/rdas/

Glycaemic Index
1. http://www.mayoclinic.org/healthy-living/nutrition-and-healthy-eating/in-depth/glycemic-index-diet/art-20048478?pg=2
2. http://www.health.harvard.edu/diseases-and-conditions/glycemic index and glycemic load for 100 foods
3. http://lpi.oregonstate.edu/infocenter/foods/grains/gigl.html

Exercise, Rest and Recreation
1. http://www.mentalhealthamerica.net/conditions/rest-relaxation-and-exercise
2. http://www.kripalu.org/article/837/

3. http://www.better-sleep-better-life.com/benefits-of-sleep.html

Health Topics

1. http://www.nlm.nih.gov/medlineplus/healthtopics.html

Quotes

1. http://www.goodreads.com/author/quotes/248774. Hippocrates
2. http://www.goodreads.com/author/quotes/657773. Jim Rohn
3. www.manifestintuition.com/body-quotes.html

Appendices

Appendix 1
Your Daily Calorie Requirement

In any meal planning exercise to achieve the goals set, the single most important factor is calories - more specifically, the total daily calorie intake.

- Eat more than you burn and chances are that you will put on weight.
- Eat less than you burn and chances are that you will slim down.
- Eat as much as you burn and your weight is likely to be steady.

It is a case of simple arithmetic.

For planning your meals, you do need to make some simple calculations to guide us. The calculations are related to the total calories that you should consume in a day to obtain the results that you want.

The basic formulae are:

For Weight Loss
Calculating Our Total Daily Metabolic Requirements
Basal Metabolic Rate
+ Caloric Intake for Exercise
= Actual Daily Caloric Requirement
Minus 300 calories for slow Weight Loss or 500 calories for Fast Weight Loss
= Daily Meals Caloric Maximum
To meet your objectives, this is the caloric intake for the day.

For Weight Gain
Calculating Our Total Daily Metabolic Requirements
Basal Metabolic Rate
+ Caloric Intake for Exercise
= Actual Daily Caloric Requirement
X 2 for Weight Gain Program
= Daily Meals Caloric Maximum
To meet your objectives, this is the caloric intake for the day.

Formulae for Calculating Total Metabolic Rate
The formula to calculate the TMR for a person who *does not exercise* at all is:
Resting Metabolic Rate (RMR) = BMR reading from Tanita Scan
Active Metabolic Rate (AMR) = BMR x 0.30 (for Men) or BMR x 0.25 (for Ladies)
For a person who does no exercise at all,
TMR = BMR x 1.30 for men or BMR x 1.25 for Ladies
For a *person who exercises*, you need to factor in the type of exercise. For example:
Light Exercise (aerobics, jogging, weights) uses up 200 calories/hour
Heavy Exercise (basketball, soccer, swimming) uses up 300 calories/hour.
If this person does light exercise, e.g. jogging, 3 times weekly, the additional weekly calorie requirement would be 200 calories x 3 = 600 calories. The additional daily calorie requirement would be 600 calories/7 days = 85.7 calories/day.

Say that there are 3 friends – John, Jane and Bob. Their current health statistics are as follows:

Current Health Status

	Particulars	John	Jane	Bob
1	Age	30	27	21
2	Gender	Male	Female	Male
3	Height	183 cm	170 cm	183 cm
4	Weight	95 kg	55 kg	83 kg
5	Body fat %	26	22	16
6	Visceral Fat	12	5	8

From their respective height, their ideal weight is easily calculated The formula to calculate the ideal weight for a man is to take his actual height (in cms) and subtract 100 from it. The formula to calculate the ideal weight for a lady is to take her actual height (in cms) and subtract 110 from it.

Weight Management

	Particulars	John	Jane	Bob
1	Age	30	27	21
2	Gender	Male	Female	Male
3	Height	183 cm	170 cm	183 cm
4	Weight	95 kg	55 kg	83 kg
5	Body fat %	26	22	16
6	Visceral Fat	12	5	8
7	Ideal Weight	83 kgs	60 kgs	83 kgs
8	**Weight Adj.**	**-12 kgs**	**+5 kgs**	**0 kgs**
9	Recommended Meal Plan	TBD*	TBD*	TBD*

TBD* = To Be determined

Total Metabolic Rate Calculation

Item	Description	Abbr.	John	Jane
1	BMR Reading	BMR	1,900	1,400
2	Active Metabolic Rate (0.30 for men; 0.25 for ladies)	AMR	510	425
3	BMR + AMR (before exercise)		2,410	1,825
4	Exercise (jogging) (3 times weekly) (200 * 3)/7	EXC	-	86
5	Total Metabolic Rate (Item 3 + Item 4)	TMR	**2,410**	**1,911**
6	Adjustment for weight gain/loss or weight maintenance program	WG/WL or WM Program	???	???
7	Recommended Meal Plan		To be determined	To be determined

John needs to lose 12 kgs of body fat; Jane is too skinny and has to put on 5 kgs of muscle; Bob is in the ideal weight range for his height.

Before any plan can be drawn up to help each person achieve their weight management goals, it is necessary to calculate their respective Total Metabolic Rate, given their current Basal Metabolic Rate.

John and Jane are jogging partners. They jog three times a week. Bob follows a sedentary lifestyle. Their individual Total Metabolic Rate are calculated as shown in the table below.

Total Metabolic Rate Calculation

	Particulars	John	Jane	Bob
1	Age	30	27	21
2	Gender	Male	Female	Male
3	Height	183 cm	170 cm	183 cm
4	Weight	95 kg	55 kg	83 kg
5	Body fat %	26	22	16
6	Visceral Fat	12	5	8
7	Ideal Weight	83 kgs	60 kgs	83 kgs
8	**Weight Adj.**	**-12 kgs**	**+5 kgs**	**0 kgs**
9	Recommended Meal Plan	TBD*	TBD*	TBD*
10	BMR Reading **(BMR)**	1,900	1,700	1900
11	Active Metabolic Rate **(AMR)** (0.30 for men; 0.25 for ladies)	570	425	570
12	BMR + AMR (before exercise)	2,470	2,125	2,470
13	Exercise (jogging) (3 times weekly) (200 * 3)/7	86	86	0
14	Total Metabolic Rate **(TMR)** (Item 12 + Item 13)	**2,556**	**2,211**	**2,470**

Now that the TMR for each person is known, individualised meal plans can be drawn up to guide their efforts to achieve their goals.

Additionally, John's visceral fat reading is 12; he has to bring his visceral fat reading down to the 5 – 8 range.

Jane has a visceral fat reading of 5; she needs to maintain it at this level. Bob has a visceral fat reading of 8. On the surface, it says that it is in the healthy range. But when we take his age into consideration as well (he is only 21 years old), he needs to work on bringing it down to 5. If he does not do so, this figure could easily climb up to 9 and above.

BODY COMPOSITION Apart from total weight, body composition affects health too – a person's Body Fat % and his Muscle Mass %. We need to check Bob's actual body fat % against that of a healthy person of his age. In our example, Bob's body fat % is 18; the healthy body fat % of a person in the age group is 14.5 to 18.0. In these circumstance, Bob need not do anything different. If, however, Bob's body fat % had been greater than 18, he would need to take measures to lose body fat and increase muscle mass whilst staying on his ideal weight.

Just changing the body composition (less body fat and more muscle mass) can have a positive impact on a person's health.

Appendix 2 **Getting Healthier**

Direction and Goals

For John, he has to lose body fat weight by 12 kgs. Jane has to gain lean muscle (5 kgs) and Bob is to maintain his current weight. The direction for each is clear and the goals are definitive, measurable and a timeframe for completion can be calculated using the meal plans drawn up for each of them.

Maintaining The Ideal

The other aspect for John, Jane and Bob to take note of is health maintenance. Once John and Jane have reached their ideal weight, they need to continue to keep in practice all the good habits that they have cultivated in their journey to better health. If either one abandons the good habits and reverts to their old habits, their health situation can slowly deteriorate and their hard won results can be slowly drained away. *Maintenance is key.*

The Soft Factors

The calculated targets are really good indicators; it gives the person a target to aim at and a time frame in which to do it. There is nothing worse than not having a firm target and not knowing how long it will take to achieve something – like being in a pitch black room with no light. Yet do not be fixated on absolute figures. Other "soft" factors need to be taken into consideration as well. The important "soft" factors are:

    a. How do you feel about yourself? Are you feeling great?
    b. How do you look? Amazing?

c. What is the feedback from those who love you? Is the feedback positive? Are they saying that there is no need to push any further?

If the answer to all three questions is "yes", then it is time to switch to maintenance mode. There is no need to chase the target any more. You have arrived!

Do take the "soft" factors into consideration; sometimes in your enthusiasm you may overdo things. You think you are doing the right thing when, in effect, you are not. Why?

If you lose too much body fat, you will begin to look gaunt. You can become overly muscular (unless it is your intent to really build up your body). In such a case, it becomes a new journey – one of building a new body.

Appendix 3 **Meal Planning**

In planning meals, always keep in mind the words of Hippocrates. Now what did Hippocrates say 2,500 years ago?

> "If we could give every individual the right amount of nourishment and exercise, not too little and not too much, we would have found the safest way to health."
>
> — Hippocrates

It does not matter what the objective is – lose body fat, gain muscle mass, maintain weight and/or reshape the body, the advice stands.

Remember that in terms of impact in reaching your goals, food and nutrition contributes 80%; exercise contributes the other 20 %. So do watch what you eat. You need to eat well to get the nutrients that your body requires, no matter what your goals. It is the lack of nutrients that will hinder achievement of your goals.

Case Examples

We have three scenarios to address.

- John has to lose body fat;
- Jane has to gain muscle mass;
- Bob has to maintain his weight while shedding some body fat and increasing some muscle mass.

Lose Body Fat Scenario

As calculated earlier, John has to lose 12 kgs. In body fat and he has to trim down his visceral fat. He has a TMR of 2,556.

John is only 30 years of age – a young man by any standard. Being young, he can be a little bit more ambitious in his plans to shed body fat. A young person can easily accommodate a daily meal plan that yields between 300 to 500 calories less than the TMR.

An older person (over 50 years of age) attempting to reach the same goals can plan meals that yield between 100 to 300 calories less than the TMR. It is not wise for older persons to attempt to be as ambitious as younger people.

Also note that the planned daily meal should never exceed 500 calories less than the TMR. The emphasis of the plan should be on ease and safety – easy to follow without in any way endangering the health of those following the plan.

A meal – any meal – should also be well-balanced; it needs to have all the food groups in the correct proportions to keep the body healthy. A meal that is not balanced – one that replaces one food group over another e.g. only proteins without carbohydrates, or vice-versa, can never be as good as one that has all the food groups.

Each food group has its own specific functions; denying the body any one food group is never a good solution. You may, for a short period, eat more of one food group over another, depending on your goals. This would be the loading dose - to help you get over the hump, so to speak. But you should revert to balanced meals in the shortest possible time.

Recommended Meal Plan
2,100 Calories Per Day

Meal	Time	Food	Cals
Breakfast	7.00 a m	Protein Shake & Oats + Banana	150
Mid-morn	10.00 a m	1 Banana or Apple	100
Lunch	1.00 p m	1 Bowl Rice/Veg	200
		2 Chicken or Fish	600
Tea	4.00 p m	Protein Shake with Non-fat Milk or Low Sugar Soya Milk	150
Dinner	6.00 p m	1 Bowl Rice/Veg	200
		2 Chicken or Fish	600
Night Snack	10.00 p m	1 Banana or Apple	100
		Total Calories	**2100**

John has to shed 12 kgs. His TMR is 2,556; the planned meals for the day yield 2,100. His calorie intake is short of his requirement by 456 calories. His body has to burn fat to get the shortage of 456 calories daily – a safe reduction (less than 500 calories) and one that John can follow faithfully (he will not feel hungry and be tempted otherwise).

In the course of a month, he will burn 456 x 30 calories = 13,680 calories.

4,500 calories is the equivalent of 1 kg. John has to shed 12 kgs i.e. the equivalent of 54,000 calories. This will take John 54,000/13,680 = 4.0 months.

By eating less per day, John can trim down in a safe and healthy way. In the course of 4.0 months, he should be down to his ideal weight.

And do not forget to drink lots of fluids – preferably plain water or water with the 3 slices of lemon in it. Water is the cleansing agent and will greatly facilitate the flushing out of the body's metabolic wastes.

Hot Tip

In the effort to shed body fat, green apples (Granny Smiths) are particularly helpful. For your snacks, eat green apples.

Gain Weight Scenario

As calculated above, Jane has to gain 5 kgs. To gain weight is actually tougher than to lose weight. It requires that the person seeking to gain weight must eat more, eat more frequently, and eat more of the right food. This sounds like food heaven – but it is not.

Jane has a TMR of 2,211; she needs to gain 5kgs. Let us say that she follows a meal plan giving her 2,300 calories daily.

2300 – 2211 calories = surplus of 89 calories daily.

89 calories x 30 days = 2,670 calories per month.

4,500 calories make up 1 kg.

Weight gain is 2,670/4500 = 0.6 kgs. in one month.

Jane can gain the 5 kgs in 8 - 9 months. She can gain the weight even faster but it means that she has to eat more. In this case, her daily meals need to yield more than 2,300 calories daily.

Meal plans are flexible and can be adjusted to suit her needs.

Recommended Meal Plan
2,100 Calories Per Day

Meal	Time	Food	Cals
Breakfast	7.00 a m	Protein Shake & Oats + Banana	150
Mid-morn	10.00 a m	1 Banana or Apple	100
Lunch	1.00 p m	1 Bowl Rice/Veg	200
		2 Chicken or Fish	600
Tea	4.00 p m	Protein Shake with Non-fat Milk or Low Sugar Soya Milk	150
Dinner	6.00 p m	1 Bowl Rice/Veg	200
		2 Chicken or Fish	600
Night Snack	10.00 p m	1 Banana or Apple	100
		Total Calories	**2100**

The requirement to drink more fluids, especially plain water, is also applicable here.

Hot Tip - to put on more muscle mass, take more proteins. Fish is particularly good as it will also give you additional essential fatty acids.

Maintain Weight and/or Reshape Body Scenario

Two persons may be of the correct weight for the same height and yet one person could be healthier than the other. This means that the other details – body fat and muscle mass could be out of balance. The unhealthy person could be carrying an excessive amount of fat compared to the muscle mass; the other person could have both body fat and muscle mass in the healthy range. The details are just as important as the overall weight.

In Bob's case, he has to eat enough on a daily basis to maintain his weight. But he also needs to bring his body fat down and gain a little bit more muscle mass in the process. This means taking meals that are a bit more loaded with proteins than in the past.

Recommended Meal Plan

1,900 Calories Per Day

Meal	Time	Food	Cals
Breakfast	7.00 a m	Protein Shake & Oats + Banana	150
Mid-morn	10.00 a m		
Lunch	1.00 p m	1 Bowl Rice/Veg	200
		2 Chicken or Fish	600
Tea	4.00 p m	Protein Shake	

		with Non-fat Milk or Low Sugar Soya Milk	150
Dinner	7.00 p m	1 Bowl Rice/Veg	200
		2 Chicken or Fish	600
Night Snack	10.00 p m		
		Total Calories	**1900**

To reshape his body, he should go for walks 3 times a week.
The walks will help him burn some fat and build up his muscles.

Appendix 4
More Sample Meal Plans

Meal Plans Are Just Guidelines

Please bear in mind that the meals planned are guides. You are free to substitute the foods you like so long as you stay within the stipulated total calories. For example, instead of white rice, you may choose to eat brown rice; instead of potatoes, you may prefer yam. This is perfectly all right.

Where proteins are concerned, try to eat fish twice a week; if you prefer whole proteins in grain form, try quinoa seeds. Do not be afraid to make substitutes to the sample plans.

Simple Rules of Thumb

Choose the foods you love to eat – this will make following the meal plan fun and enjoyable. Just make sure that the Total Calories are not exceeded.

Buy local produce – this will be easier on your pocket.

Use produce that are in season – these are more economical.

Do not deny yourself – on occasions, you may indulge yourself to your favourite foods. Just do not over indulge and do not do it too frequently. Remember this - you should enjoy the journey, not miss out on the fun.

Portion Size – this refers to the plate that you use to hold our food. Use a smaller plate to hold your food; the smaller plate will not hold as much physically. Psychologically, when you look at the plate, it will look full to you.

Do not overeat - eat until you feel about 80% full. The moment you feel a little full, that is the time to stop eating. I have known friends who have eaten so much at lunch/dinner occasions that they had to loosen the belts/buttons of their pants! Now that is overeating by any standard.

Proportions - when planning a meal, visualise what it would look like on the plate.

- Divide the plate up into 4 quarters.
- 2 quarters (half) of the plate is for vegetables and fruits – colourful vegetables that will give you the fibre, carbohydrates and the nutrients needed.
- One quarter of the plate is reserved for carbohydrates.
- The other quarter is for protein.

The important point is to get the nutrition we need, not how full we feel.

Remember that the meals shown here are just guides to help you get started. They are not meant to be carved in stone. Adjust them to suit your taste.

The key point is to know your TMR (Total Metabolic Rate) and proceed from there.

For body fat reduction, take a plan that is 300 to 500 calories less than your TMR; make sure that this range (300 to 500 calories) does not exceed 20% of your TMR.

For muscle gain, do not try to eat too much daily.

Mohd Ilhan Abdullah

Recommended Meal Plan 1,000 Calories Per Day

Meal	Time	Food	Cals
Breakfast	7 a m	Protein Shake & Oats + Banana	150
Mid-morn	10 a m		
Lunch	1 p m	1/2 Bowl Rice/ Veg	100
		1 Chicken or Fish	300
Tea	4 p m	Protein Shake with Water	80
Dinner	7 p m	1/2 Bowl Rice/ Veg	100
		1 Chicken or Fish	300
Night Snack	10 p m		

Total Calories 1030

Recommended Meal Plan 1,100 Calories Per Day

Meal	Time	Food	Cals
Breakfast	7 a m	Protein Shake & Oats + Banana	150
Mid-morn	10 a m		
Lunch	1 p m	1 Bowl Rice/ Veg	200
		1 Chicken or Fish	300
Tea	4 p m	Protein Shake with Water	80
Dinner	7 p m	1/2 Bowl Rice/ Veg	100
		1 Chicken or Fish	300
Night Snack	10 p m		

Total Calories 1130

Meal	Time	Food	Cals	*	Meal	Time	Food	Cals
Recommended Meal Plan					**Recommended Meal Plan**			
1,200 Calories Per Day					**1,300 Calories Per Day**			
Breakfast	7 a m	Protein Shake & Oats + Banana	150	*	Breakfast	7 a m	Protein Shake & Oats + Banana	150
Mid-morn	10 a m			*	Mid-morn	10 a m		
Lunch	1 p m	1 Bowl Rice/ Veg	200	*	Lunch	1 p m	1 Bowl Rice/ Veg	200
		1 Chicken or Fish	300				1 Chicken or Fish	300
Tea	4 p m	Protein Shake		*	Tea	4 p m	Protein Shake	
		with Water	80				with Non-fat Milk	150
							or Low Sugar Soya Milk	
Dinner	7 p m	1 Bowl Rice/ Veg	200	*	Dinner	7 p m	1 Bowl Rice/ Veg	200
		1 Chicken or Fish	300				1 Chicken or Fish	300
Night Snack	10 p m			*	Night Snack	10 p m		
Total Calories			**1230**	*	**Total Calories**			**1300**

Recommended Meal Plan 1,400 Calories Per Day				*	Recommended Meal Plan 1,500 Calories Per Day			
Meal	Time	Food	Cals	*	Meal	Time	Food	Cals
Breakfast	7 a m	Protein Shake & Oats + Banana	150	*	Breakfast	7 a m	Protein Shake & Oats + Banana	150
Mid-morn	10 a m	1 Banana or Apple	100	*	Mid-morn	10 a m	1 Banana or Apple	100
Lunch	1 p m	1 Bowl Rice/ Veg	200	*	Lunch	1 p m	1 Bowl Rice/ Veg	200
		1 Chicken or Fish	300				1 Chicken or Fish	300
Tea	4 p m	Protein Shake with Non-fat Milk	150	*	Tea	4 p m	Protein Shake with Non-fat Milk	150
		or Low Sugar Soya Milk					or Low Sugar Soya Milk	
Dinner	7 p m	1 Bowl Rice/ Veg	200	*	Dinner	7 p m	1 Bowl Rice/ Veg	200
		1 Chicken or Fish	300				1 Chicken or Fish	300
Night Snack	10 p m			*	Night Snack	10 p m	1 Banana or Apple	100
		Total Calories	1400	*			Total Calories	1500

Meal	Time	Food	Cals	*	Meal	Time	Food	Cals
Recommended Meal Plan **1,600 Calories Per Day**				*	**Recommended Meal Plan** **1,700 Calories Per Day**			
Breakfast	7 a m	Protein Shake & Oats + Banana	150	*	Breakfast	7 a m	Protein Shake & Oats + Banana	150
Mid-morn	10 a m			*	Mid-morn	10 a m	1 Banana or Apple	100
Lunch	1 p m	1 Bowl Rice/ Veg 2 Chicken or Fish	200 600	*	Lunch	1 p m	1 Bowl Rice/ Veg 2 Chicken or Fish	200 600
Tea	4 p m	Protein Shake with Non-fat Milk or Low Sugar Soya Milk	150	*	Tea	4 p m	Protein Shake with Non-fat Milk or Low Sugar Soya Milk	150
Dinner	7 p m	1 Bowl Rice/ Veg 1 Chicken or Fish	200 300	*	Dinner	7 p m	1 Bowl Rice/ Veg 1 Chicken or Fish	200 300
Night Snack	10 p m			*	Night Snack	10 p m		
		Total Calories	**1600**	*			**Total Calories**	**1700**

Mohd Ilhan Abdullah

Recommended Meal Plan 1,800 Calories Per Day

Meal	Time	Food	Cals
Breakfast	7 a m	Protein Shake & Oats + Banana	150
Mid-morn	10 a m	1 Banana or Apple	100
Lunch	1 p m	1 Bowl Rice/ Veg	200
		2 Chicken or Fish	600
Tea	4 p m	Protein Shake with Non-fat Milk	150
		or Low Sugar Soya Milk	
Dinner	7 p m	1 Bowl Rice/ Veg	200
		1 Chicken or Fish	300
Night Snack	10 p m	1 Banana or Apple	100
		Total Calories	1800

Recommended Meal Plan 1,900 Calories Per Day

Meal	Time	Food	Cals
Breakfast	7 a m	Protein Shake & Oats + Banana	150
Mid-morn	10 a m		
Lunch	1 p m	1 Bowl Rice/ Veg	200
		2 Chicken or Fish	600
Tea	4 p m	Protein Shake with Non-fat Milk	150
		or Low Sugar Soya Milk	
Dinner	7 p m	1 Bowl Rice/ Veg	200
		2 Chicken or Fish	600
Night Snack	10 p m		
		Total Calories	1900

Meal	Time	Food	Cals	*	Meal	Time	Food	Cals
Breakfast	7 a m	Protein Shake & Oats + Banana	150	*	Breakfast	7 a m	Protein Shake & Oats + Banana	150
Mid-morn	10 a m	1 Banana or Apple	100	*	Mid-morn	10 a m	1 Banana or Apple	100
Lunch	1 p m	1 Bowl Rice/ Veg	200	*	Lunch	1 p m	1 Bowl Rice/ Veg	200
		2 Chicken or Fish	600				2 Chicken or Fish	600
Tea	4 p m	Protein Shake with Non-fat Milk	150	*	Tea	4 p m	Protein Shake with Non-fat Milk	150
		or Low Sugar Soya Milk					or Low Sugar Soya Milk	
Dinner	7 p m	1 Bowl Rice/ Veg	200	*	Dinner	7 p m	1 Bowl Rice/ Veg	200
		2 Chicken or Fish	600				2 Chicken or Fish	600
Night Snack	10 p m			*	Night Snack	10 p m	1 Banana or Apple	100

Recommended Meal Plan 2,000 Calories Per Day (left) — **Total Calories 2000**

Recommended Meal Plan 2,100 Calories Per Day (right) — **Total Calories 2100**

Recommended Meal Plan
2,300 Calories Per Day

Meal	Time	Food	Cals
Breakfast	7 a m	Protein Shake & Oats + Banana	150
Mid-morn	10 a m	1 Banana or Apple	100
Lunch	1 p m	2 Bowl Rice/Veg	400
		2 Chicken or Fish	600
Tea	4 p m	Protein Shake with Non-fat Milk or Low Sugar Soya Milk	150
Dinner	7 p m	1 Bowl Rice/Veg	200
		2 Chicken or Fish	600
Night Snack	10 p m	1 Banana or Apple	100
		Total Calories	**2300**

Recommended Meal Plan
2,500 Calories Per Day

Meal	Time	Food	Cals
Breakfast	7 a m	Protein Shake & Oats + Banana	150
Mid-morn	10 a m	1 Banana or Apple	100
Lunch	1 p m	2 Bowl Rice/Veg	400
		2 Chicken or Fish	600
Tea	4 p m	Protein Shake with Non-fat Milk or Low Sugar Soya Milk	150
Dinner	7 p m	2 Bowl Rice/Veg	400
		2 Chicken or Fish	600
Night Snack	10 p m	1 Banana or Apple	100
		Total Calories	**2500**